D0922618

Minimally Invasive Surgery in Orthopedics

Giles R. Scuderi • Alfred J. Tria

Editors

Minimally Invasive Surgery in Orthopedics

Knee Handbook

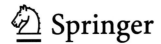

Editors
Giles R. Scuderi, MD
Insall Scott Kelly Institute
for Orthopaedics and Sports Medicine
New York, NY, USA
grscuderi@aol.com

Alfred J. Tria, Jr., MD
Department of Orthopaedic Surgery
UMDNJ-Robert Wood Johnson Hospital
One Robert Wood Johnson Place
New Brunswick, NJ 08903-0019
atriajrmd@aol.com

ISBN 978-1-4614-0678-5   e-ISBN 978-1-4614-0679-2
DOI 10.1007/978-1-4614-0679-2
Springer New York Dordrecht Heidelberg London

Library of Congress Control Number: 2011937226

© Springer Science+Business Media, LLC 2012
All rights reserved. This work may not be translated or copied in whole or in part without the
written permission of the publisher (Springer Science+Business Media, LLC, 233 Spring
Street, New York, NY 10013, USA), except for brief excerpts in connection with reviews or
scholarly analysis. Use in connection with any form of information storage and retrieval,
electronic adaptation, computer software, or by similar or dissimilar methodology now
known or hereafter developed is forbidden.
The use in this publication of trade names, trademarks, service marks, and similar terms, even if
they are not identified as such, is not to be taken as an expression of opinion as to whether or not
they are subject to proprietary rights.
While the advice and information in this book are believed to be true and accurate at the date
of going to press, neither the authors nor the editors nor the publisher can accept any legal
responsibility for any errors or omissions that may be made. The publisher makes no warranty,
express or implied, with respect to the material contained herein.

Printed on acid-free paper

Springer is part of Springer Science+Business Media (www.springer.com)

Contents

Contributors

Rodney K. Alan, MD Attending Surgeon, Department of Surgery, Saint Peter's University Hospital, New Brunswick, NJ, USA

Richard A. Berger, MD Assistant Professor, Department of Orthopaedic Surgery, Rush-Presbyterian-St. Luke's Medical Center, Chicago, IL, USA

Eddie Bibbiani, MD Attending Surgeon, Centro Chirurgia Protesica, Istituto Ortopedico "R. Galeazzi,", Milan, Italy

Peter Bonutti, MD Founder and CEO, Associate Clinical Professor, Bonutti Clinic, Effingham, IL, USA

Department of Orthopaedics, University of Arkansas, Little Rock, AR, USA

Nicolò Castelnuovo, MD Attending Surgeon, Centro Chirurgia Protesica, Istituto Ortopedico "R. Galeazzi,", Milan, Italy

F. d'Amario, MD Attending Surgeon, Centro Chirurgia Protesica, Istituto Ortopedico "R. Galeazzi,", Milan, Italy

Steven B. Haas, MD, MPH Chief of Knee Service, Associate Professor, Department of Orthopedic Surgery, Hospital for Special Surgery, New York, NY, USA

Weill Medical College of Cornell University, New York, NY, USA

Richard H. Hallock, MD CEO, The Orthopedic Institute of Pennsylvania, Camp Hill, PA, USA

Jodi F. Hartman, MS President, Orthopaedic Research & Reporting, Ltd., Gahanna, OH, USA

Peter F. Heeckt, MD Chief Medical Officer, Smith & Nephew, Inc, Memphis, TN, USA

Mohanjit Kochhar, MD Attending Surgeon, North Middlesex University Hospital, London, UK

Jess H. Lonner, MD Director, Knee Replacement Surgery, Director, Orthopaedic Research, Booth Bartolozzi Balderston Orthopaedics, Pennsylvania Hospital, Philadelphia, PA, USA

Samuel J. Macdessi, MBBS (Hons), FRACS Staff, Sydney Knee
Specialists, Edgecliff, Australia

Sabine Mai, MD Attending Orthopaedic Surgeon,
Kassel Orthopaedic Center, Kassel, Germany

Mary Ann Manitta, RN Clinical Nurse, Department of Orthopedics,
Hospital for Special Surgery, New York, NY, USA

Mark W. Pagnano, MD Associate Professor, Department of Orthopaedic
Surgery, Mayo Clinic College of Medicine, Mayo Clinic,
Rochester, MN, USA

John A. Repicci, DDS, MD Private Practice, Joint Reconstruction
Orthopedic Center, Buffalo, NY, USA

Sergio Romagnoli, MD Attending Surgeon, Centro Chirurgia Protesica,
Istituto Ortopedico "R. Galeazzi,", Milan, Italy

Aaron G. Rosenberg, MD Professor, Department of Orthopaedic
Surgery, Rush Medical College, Rush-Presbyterian-St. Luke's
Medical Center, Chicago, IL, USA

Paul L. Saenger, MD Private Practice, Blue Ridge Bone & Joint Clinic,
PA, Asheville, NC, USA

Giles R. Scuderi, MD, FACS Director, Attending Orthopedic Surgeon,
Assistant Clinical Professor of Orthopedic Surgery, Insall Scott Kelly
Institute for Orthopaedics and Sports Medicine, New York, NY, USA

North Shore-LIJ Health System, Great Neck, NY, USA

Albert Einstein College of Medicine, New York, NY, USA

Werner Siebert, MD Professor of Orthopaedic Surgery and Chairman,
Kassel Orthopaedic Center, Kassel, Germany

James B. Stiehl, MD Clinical Associate Professor,
Department of Orthopaedic Surgery, Medical College of Wisconsin,
Milwaukee, WI, USA

S. David Stulberg, MD Clinical Professor,
Department of Orthopaedic Surgery, Feinberg School of Medicine,
Northwestern University, Chicago, IL, USA

Alfred J. Tria Jr., MD Department of Orthopaedic Surgery,
UMDNJ-Robert Wood Johnson Hospital, One Robert Wood Johnson Place,
New Brunswick, NJ, USA

Department of Orthopedic Surgery, Robert Wood Johnson Medical School,
Piscataway, NJ, USA

Francesco Verde, MD Attending Surgeon, Centro Chirurgia Protesica,
Istituto Ortopedico "R. Galeazzi,", Milan, Italy

MIS Unicondylar Arthroplasty: The Bone-Sparing Technique

John A. Repicci and Jodi F. Hartman

Minimally invasive (MIS) unicondylar knee arthroplasty (UKA) and total knee arthroplasty (TKA) each have specific indications and distinctive roles in the senior author's algorithm for the treatment of knee osteoarthritis (OA). MIS UKA is not a substitute for TKA, which is the procedure of choice for treatment of advanced stages of OA. This philosophy is supported by Thornhill and Scott, who assert that UKA should be considered in the "continuum of surgical options for the treatment of the osteoarthritic patient" [1]. In cases of earlier, nonadvanced OA, the two procedures may act in conjunction with one another, with MIS UKA serving as a supplement to future TKA. Together, these devices may be considered as a "knee prosthetic system" [2].

With the limited survivorship of TKA and the aging of the active baby boomer population, there is a need for a procedure in addition to TKA to address the treatment of earlier, nonadvanced stages of OA and to extend the survivability of knee prosthetics. Because the knee prosthetics have a finite life span, a single device cannot encompass the entire spectrum of survivability necessary for many patients. Under the senior author's serial replacement concept, a procedure

such as MIS UKA performed at an earlier age, before TKA use and as a supplement to TKA, will absorb approximately 10 years of functional capacity so that when and if future arthroplasty is required, the survivability of the entire knee prosthetic system is lengthened [2, 3].

Minimally Invasive UKA Program

A unique feature of this serial replacement philosophy is the MIS UKA program that was introduced by the senior author in 1992 [4]. This program is significantly different from simply the use of a small incision or implementation of a MIS surgical approach. Instead, it combines the following MIS concepts into a single program.

Adjunct Use of Arthroscopy

This multipronged MIS approach begins with arthroscopic evaluation prior to arthroplasty, which allows assessment of the articular cartilage in the contralateral compartment and permits the evaluation of the contralateral meniscus. The contralateral meniscus cannot be visualized through traditional surgical exposure alone. If the contralateral compartment has advanced OA or if the contralateral meniscus is not intact, the preplanned MIS UKA procedure may be abandoned in favor of TKA.

Verification of a fully functioning, intact, contralateral meniscus is critical for successful UKA,

J.A. Repicci (✉)
Private Practice, Joint Reconstruction Orthopedic Center,
Buffalo, NY, USA
e-mail: repicci@adelphia.net

J.F. Hartman
Orthopaedic Research & Reporting, Ltd.,
Gahanna, OH, USA

G.R. Scuderi and A.J. Tria (eds.), *Minimally Invasive Surgery in Orthopedics: Knee Handbook*,
DOI 10.1007/978-1-4614-0679-2_1, © Springer Science+Business Media, LLC 2012

as the load-bearing surface area and the stability of the knee joint are enhanced by intact menisci [5–11]. Due to the lower tibiofemoral contact area compared with TKA designs, a certain degree of cold flow is permissible in UKA designs, but an absent contralateral meniscus will result in an inadequate amount of tibiofemoral contact. If UKA is performed in spite of an absent contralateral meniscus, the continued osteoarthritic progression may hasten the rate of degeneration of the untreated contralateral side, possibly leading to early failure of the UKA device [12]. Thus, although eliminating overcorrection has reduced the incidence of UKA failures in recent years [1, 6, 12–25], contralateral compartment degeneration and early UKA failure remain a concern if the contralateral meniscus is not intact and the cruciate ligaments are not properly balanced.

Minimally Invasive Surgical Approach Avoiding Patellar Dislocation

A distinction must be made between a MIS surgical approach and a "mini incision," which merely is a small hole and may result in significant distortion of soft tissue. A MIS surgical approach requires preservation of all possible tissues required for any future restoration, including the suprapatellar pouch, the quadriceps tendon, the patella, and the medial tibial buttress. The only UKA system meeting these criteria is the MIS bone-sparing UKA technique. By combining UKA with a MIS surgical approach, a reduction in postoperative morbidity and pain, a decrease in rehabilitation time without the need for formal physical therapy, and the ability to perform the procedure on a same-day or short-stay basis are possible [4, 26–31]. Compared with traditional open UKA, MIS UKA is associated with faster rates of recovery and earlier discharge [29, 30, 32]. In addition, equal reliability, without compromising proper component placement or long-term survivorship, has been demonstrated between a MIS surgical approach and a wide incision [26, 29, 32]. The diminished postoperative pain and decreased rehabilitation time associated with MIS UKA most likely is a

result of preservation of the quadriceps tendon and not the short skin incision itself [32].

Resurfacing UKA Design with Inlay Tibial Component

Another key feature of the senior author's MIS UKA program is the use of a resurfacing UKA design with an inlay tibial component. A significant problem in the conversion of UKA to TKA is medial tibial bone loss [33, 34]. The use of an all-polyethylene inlay tibial component requires minimal bone resection and preserves the medial buttress and, therefore, is advantageous compared with use of their modular, saw-cut tibial counterparts, which are thicker and require significantly more bone resection. Due to the minimally invasive nature of the bone-sparing UKA technique, conversion to a TKA may be considered as a delayed primary TKA. An additional source of bone resection with other UKA systems is the full exposure often required for jig instrumentation. Finally, because many saw-cut tibial designs employ peg or fin fixation, tibial bone is further compromised upon implant removal and may necessitate the use as bone grafts, special custom devises, or metal wedge tibial trays to stabilize the tibia during conversion to TKA [33–37].

Pain Management with Local Anesthetic and Without Use of Narcotics

Outpatient status is possible with the advocated MIS UKA program due to a structure pain management protocol. Spinal or general anesthesia is used in all cases. During surgery, 30 mg ketorolac tromethamine (15 mg for patients older than 65 years of age) is administered either intramuscularly or intravenously and is repeated after 5 h in patients with normal renal function. All incised tissues are infiltrated with long-acting local anesthetics to further pain relief. Additional components of the pain management protocol include patient education, avoidance of cerebral-depressing injectable narcotics, and the preemptive use of scheduled oral 400 mg ibuprofen every 4 h and oral 500 mg acetaminophen/5 mg hydrocodone bitartrate every 4 h for the first 3 days postoperatively.

As a result of this multimodal pain management program, patients are fully alert in the recovery room and have no local knee pain. Because pain is absent, the patients are able to perform straight leg raises and to actively participate in the postoperative rehabilitation process. The use of anesthetic and avoidance of narcotics are credited for shortening the recovery and rehabilitation time, permitting the procedure to be performed on an outpatient basis.

Patient Selection

Proper patient selection is a significant factor contributing to the success of UKA for both MIS and traditional techniques. According to the senior author's selection criteria, all patients between 50 and 90 years of age who are diagnosed with OA, have failed nonoperative treatment, present with weight-bearing pain that significantly impairs quality of life, and have weight-bearing radiographs with complete loss of medial joint space are considered candidates for MIS UKA. During the preoperative evaluation, radiographic assessment identifies pathological changes and establishes the extent of OA; physical examination determines the degree of pain, function, and deformity; and patient discussion divulges activities of daily living limitations, as well as occupational and functional demands, which are of particular importance in electing UKA [17, 38]. Although this preoperative evaluation assists in selecting potential UKA candidates, the decision to perform UKA may only be finalized at the time of surgery, at which point the status of the contralateral compartment and meniscus are evaluated.

A thorough radiographic analysis is critical to the patient selection process. In addition to obtaining weight-bearing anteroposterior, lateral, and patellofemoral radiographs, the Ahlback classification routinely is used to grade the progression of medial compartment OA [39]. The anatomic tibiofemoral alignment averages 6° varus for medial disease [40]. To qualify for UKA, OA must be confined to a single tibiofemoral compartment on weight-bearing radiograph. According to Sisto et al., the key to UKA success is being absolutely certain that OA is confined only to the involved compartment that is to be replaced [41]. Slight degenerative changes in the contralateral compartment, however, may be permissible and do not seem to adversely affect the results of UKA provided that the articular cartilage on the weight-bearing surface of the contralateral compartment appears adequate [15, 20, 21, 42, 43]. The presence of large osteophytes on the femoral condyle of the uninvolved compartment, however, may be indicative of bi- or tri-compartmental disease and, hence, is a contraindication to UKA [1, 20, 44].

Because the joint line becomes elevated by several millimeters in the weight-bearing position, most patients with medial OA exhibit an altered patellofemoral compartment, which is not considered a contraindication for UKA [20, 21, 42]. UKA should not be an option, however, if the Merchant's view demonstrates sclerosis with marked loss of lateral patellofemoral joint space [40].

Although the majority of patients selected for UKA demonstrate Ahlback stage 2 (absence of joint line) or stage 3 (minor bone attrition), the procedure may be considered in selected cases with Ahlback stage 4 (moderate bone attrition) [40]. Patients with Ahlback stage 1 should be excluded from consideration, as the disease progression is in its early stages. Ahlback stage 5 patients have advanced OA with gross bone attrition, and, therefore, are more appropriately treated with TKA [40].

For Ahlback stage 2, 3, and 4 patients to be considered as UKA candidates, range of motion must be at least 10–90° [2, 3]. Instability, such as a compromised anterior cruciate ligament (ACL), is a relative contraindication to medial UKA [1–3, 23, 43, 45–47], but an absolute contraindication to lateral UKA [2, 3]. Rheumatoid arthritis, extensive avascular necrosis, and active or recent infection are absolute contraindications [2, 3]. As long as absolute indications are met, certain relative contraindications, including obesity and high activity, do not appear to significantly affect UKA survivorship [22, 25, 47].

Whereas other surgeons adhere to strict selection criteria [18, 48–50], concentrating on absolute indications and contraindications, the senior author follows a broad approach [3, 31], considering patient choice rather than definitive criteria. In accordance to the serial replacement concept, MIS UKA is used to treat patients with unicompartmental OA who wish to avoid or postpone TKA. If TKA is required in the future, the UKA may be converted to a primary TKA, which may survive the duration of the patient's life.

In the senior author's 25 year of offering MIS UKA, patients with unilateral OA readily accept the concept of a temporizing arthritis bypass to delay or prevent TKA. When presented with a choice between UKA and TKA, patients tend to opt for the less invasive procedure [3, 31]. In a study by Hawker et al. assessing the need for and willingness to undergo arthroplasty, less than 15% of patients with severe arthritis were definitely willing to undergo arthroplasty, which lead to the conclusion that patients' preferences and surgical indications must be considered mutually when evaluating the need and appropriateness of arthroplasty [51]. Because most patients with unicompartmental OA are inconvenienced b pain, but remain involved in recreational or professional interest, UKA is an appealing alternative to TKA as a means of not only reducing symptoms, but also of allowing continued participation in their desired activities.

Preoperative Discussion and Informed Patient Consent

A comprehensive preoperative discussion is an integral component of this treatment approach. The serial replacement concept must be explained to the patient so that he or she understands that most knee prosthetics, including UKA and primary TKA devices, have a finite survivorship. If MIS UKA is selected, the patient must be aware that it may be the first component of a serial knee prosthetic system that will be used to treat knee OA. This is of particular importance to the young, heavier, or more active patient, who must be

advised that the effectiveness of his or her UKA may be shorter than the 10-year duration experience by the average UKA patient [31, 52, 53]. Conversely, UKA in an older or less active patient may function well beyond 10 years [31, 52]. Finally, the surgeon should explain that the most appropriate treatment option, UKA or TKA, will be determined at the time of surgery. Because of the possibility of performing TKA if OA is too advanced, all patients scheduled to undergo surgery should be encouraged to sign informed consents for both UKA and TKA [1, 54].

MIS Bone-Sparing UKA Surgical Techniques

The MIS bone-sparing UKA surgical technique has been previously described [2, 4, 40, 55]. The technique for medial implantation is summarized below, as medial compartment OA is the most common indication for UKA. The goal of the procedure is to replace the medial tibiofemoral compartment and balance the forces so that body weight is equally dispersed between the replaced compartment and the opposite compartment.

Patient Preparation

General, spinal, or regional anesthesia may be employed; however, the anesthesia team must be cognizant of the goal for outpatient or short-stay rehabilitation, which require walking within 2–4 h postsurgery. Patient preparation is performed per standard protocols, with patient placement in a supine position. A thigh holder with an arterial tourniquet set at 300 mmHg is used to secure the leg. A standard operating table is used, with the foot end of the table placed in a flexed position. The MIS surgical approach requires continuous repositioning of the knee to optimize visualization, as certain structures are better visualized at low or high degrees of flexion. Because knee positioning from 0° to 120° of flexion is necessary, the lower leg and knee are drape-free.

Diagnostic Arthroscopy

Prior to commencing MIS UKA, the preoperative diagnosis of unicompartmental OA is confirmed through arthroscopy using a medial portal. In addition to verifying that the contralateral compartment is unaffected, the status of the contralateral meniscus must be inspected, as it cannot be visualized through the flexion gap during the open procedure. The extent of medial compartment damage and the status of the ACL also should be noted.

The UKA procedure should proceed only if the OA is limited to one tibiofemoral compartment and the contralateral meniscus is functional. If the disease process is more progressive, the surgeon must be prepared to perform a TKA, the potential of which should be preoperatively discussed and consented to by the patient.

Exposure with Posterior Femoral Condyle Resection

To proceed with the MIS UKA, a limited 7- to 10-cm skin incision is developed from the superomedial edge of the patella to the proximal tibial region, incorporating the arthroscopic portal. A subcutaneous dissection, producing a 2- to 5-cm skin flap surrounding the entire incision, improves skin mobility and visualization.

A medial parapatellar capsular arthrotomy is created from the superior pole of the patella to the tibia. A 2-cm transverse release of the vastus medialis tendon further enhances visualization. If additional exposure to the femoral condyle is required, a 2- to 3-cm segment of the medial parapatellar osteophyte may be resected with a sagittal saw. This medial parapatellar capsular arthrotomy is fundamental to the MIS surgical technique, as it does not violate the extensor mechanism nor does it dislocate the patella. By avoiding patellar dislocation, the suprapatellar pouch remains intact and able to unfold the required four times in length during knee flexion to 90°.[40,5,56] On the contrary, during traditional open TKA or UKA procedures, the suprapatellar pouch is damaged when the patella is everted, necessitating extensive physical therapy to reverse the iatrogenic damage.

Because the medial compartment OA is an extension gap disease (Fig. 1.1), with no defect in flexion gap, approximately 10 mm of space must be created in the flexion gap to accommodate the prosthesis. The first step in generating this space is a 5- to 8-mm resection of the posterior femoral condyle. The articular defect is located at the distal femur and the anterior tibia. An area of preserved articular cartilage, located by flexing the knee 90°, causing the femur to roll back onto the tibia, serves as an excellent reference point for reconstruction (Fig. 1.2). Curved distractor pins are inserted at the femoral and tibial levels to allow placement of a joint distractor, which improves visualization of the tibial plateau. At the posterior tibia, adjacent to the posterior tibial rim, a high-speed bur is buried 5 mm into normal cartilage to create the additional 4–5 mm of space in the flexion gap necessary for prosthetic insertion. In the anterior tibial region, corresponding to the area of articular cartilage loss and sclerotic bone formation, the medial tibial buttress is preserved by burying the bur at half-depth (3 mm). The bur holes are connected, creating a guide slot (Fig. 1.3).

During tibial resection, it is also critical to preserve a 2- to 3-mm circumferential rim, which aids in component stabilization. This entire resection process creates a bed for the all-polyethylene tibial inlay component. The natural location of femoral weight transfer at the anterior tibial level is indicated by the use of a crosshatch. The tibia inlay component then is fitted and adjusted as necessary.

Preservation of the layer of sclerotic bone creates a stable platform for the tibial component and minimizes medial tibial bone loss, which is a major cause of UKA revision [33, 34]. The importance of preserving this medical tibial buttress is analogous to the preservation of the posterior acetabular rim in total hip arthroplasty in that, if absent, future reconstruction is severely compromised. The use of resurfacing UKA designs with tibial inlay components is advantageous compared with the use of other UKA designs that require saw-cut resections and, hence, sacrifice the valuable layer of sclerotic bone, i.e., the medial tibial buttress (Fig. 1.4).

Extension Gap Disease

a   Flexion Gap   b   Extension Gap
     No ligament imbalance   ACL and MCL laxity

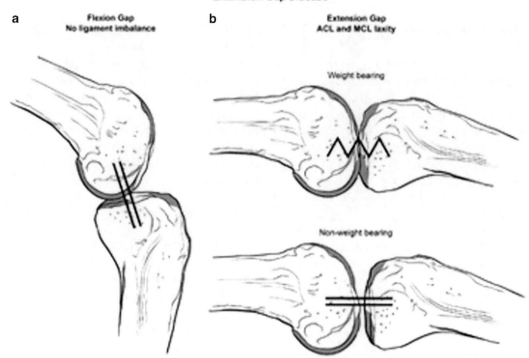

Fig. 1.1 Medial unicompartmental osteoarthritis is an extension gap disease. (**a**) No articular surface loss is present in the flexion gap. (**b**) In contrast, approximately 5 mm of articular surface is lost in the extension gap. This narrowing of the medial compartment joint space is evident on radiographic evaluation and is responsible for many of the clinical observations characteristic of medial unicompartmental osteoarthritis, including ACL and medical collateral ligament (MCL) laxity, lateral tibial thrust, or varus deformity, present in the extension gap; and absence of deformity in the flexion gap

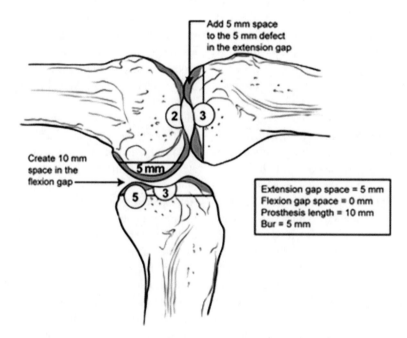

Fig. 1.2 Illustration depicting the creation of several internal landmarks, which assist in the necessary femoral and tibial resections

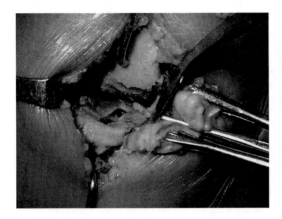

Fig. 1.3 Creation of a guide slot for tibial component insertion

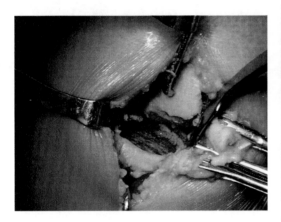

Fig. 1.4 Final preparation of the tibia. Unlike polyethylene saw-cut tibial components that require more aggressive bone resection, the use of an all-polyethylene inlay tibial component allows limited bone resection with preservation of the medial tibial buttress

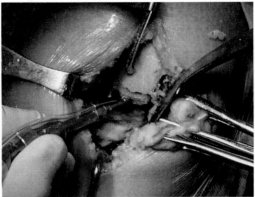

Fig. 1.5 Femoral preparation and resection

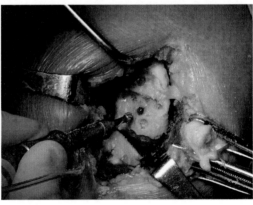

Fig. 1.6 Creation of drill hole guides to aid in femoral resection

This method of femoral resection allows adequate space for component insertion, while preventing settling.

Femoral Preparation and Resection

Femoral preparation begins by creating a depth gauge using a 5.5-mm round bur drilled to a half-depth of 3 mm into the femoral extension gap surface (Figs. 1.2 and 1.5). An additional full-depth of 5 mm is created at the junction with the previous saw cut and the distal femoral surface, which will allow the curved portion of the femoral component to set midway between the flexion and extension gaps (45° flexion position). Four 3-mm drill-hole guides are created and bulk bone is resected to the guide depth (Fig. 1.6).

Femoral-Tibial Alignment

With the knee in full extension and flexion, methylene blue marks are created on the sclerotic tibial bone and on the corresponding area of the femoral condyle to indicate both the desired center of rotation, or contact point, of the femoral component in relation to the tibial component and the desired center point of the femoral component (Fig. 1.7). A femoral drill guide with a large central slot to visualize component alignment is inserted to assist in the creation of a center femoral dill hole.

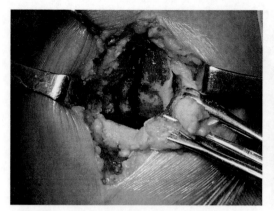

Fig. 1.7 Femoral-tibial alignment

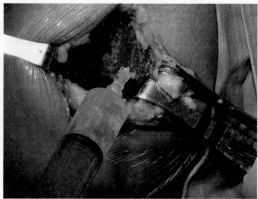

Fig. 1.8 Local anesthetic injection

Referencing the methylene blue markings, a keel-slot for the fin of the femoral component is created using a sagittal saw or side-cutting bur. The trial femoral component is placed using the femoral inserter.

Trial Reduction and Local Anesthetic Injection

Trial reduction is performed to evaluate range of motion through 115° of flexion and to assess soft tissue balancing. Lack of complete extension or flexion indicates inadequate tibial or femoral preparations. Insertion and proper alignment of appropriately sized implants should result in ligament balancing. If, however, the ligaments are tight only in the extension gap, tension may be adjusted by further bone removal at the distal femoral level. If tension is present in both the flexion and extension gaps, additional tibial bone may be resected, as previously described, in 1-mm increments until proper tension is achieved.

After satisfactory range of motion and proper soft tissue balancing are achieved, the trial components are removed, the joint is irrigated thoroughly, and a dry field is established. At this stage, both the femoral and tibial preparations are visible. Prior to component insertion, all incised tissues are infiltrated with anesthesia (0.25% bupivacaine and 0.5% epinephrine solution) for postoperative pain relief and hemostasis (Fig. 1.8).

Component Insertion and Final Preparation

After irrigation with pulse lavage and antibiotic solution, methylmethacrylate cement is used to insert all components into gauze-dried bone (Fig. 1.9). To dry the field and to aid in cement removal, sponge packs are placed in the suprapatellar pouch, posterior to the femoral condyle, and on the femoral and tibial surfaces. Excess cement is removed from the posterior recess and perimeter of the tibial component after insertion, but before femoral component placement, using a narrow nerve hook. After femoral component placement, excess cement is removed from the perimeter using a dental pick. Range of motion is performed following final prosthetic implantation to evaluate the flexion-extension gaps. Cement is cured with the knee in full extension. After the cement mantle has hardened, any remaining osteophytes should be removed. Patella contouring or notchplasty also may be performed, if necessary. As a final step, the joint is thoroughly irrigated with sterile saline.

The tourniquet is deflated and hemostasis is achieved with electrocautery. A tube drain is inserted into the contralateral component via a stab wound. Capsular closure is performed with size 0 Vicryl suture (Ethicon Company; Somerville, NJ). Subcuticular size 0 Prolene suture and sterile dressing is used for skin closure. Before exiting the operating room, a circumferential

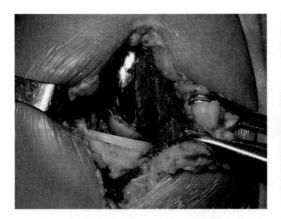

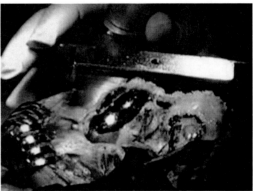

Fig. 1.9 Implantation of the UKA resurfacing prosthesis

Fig. 1.10 Femoral preparation during conversion of a UKA to a delayed primary TKA. The distal femoral is resected at 9 mm, taking care to resect all bone visible around the femoral component and undermining the bone adjacent to the fin

ice cuff, a pneumatic compression device and an immobilizer are applied.

Surgical Technique for Conversion of MIS Bone-Sparing UKA to TKA

UKA Prosthesis Removal

The Repicci II unicondylar knee system (Biomet Inc., Warsaw, IN) is designed to extend the life of a natural knee, while preserving bone. As OA advances into the lateral femoral condyle, which may occur 10 years after the UKA procedure, conversion to TKA may be necessary. The MIS nature of this particular UKA design, along with the surgical technique described below for the removal of the UKA prosthetic system, results in minimal bone loss. Because resections equivalent to those performed in a primary TKA are produced, this conversion to a TKA may be considered as a delayed primary TKA.

Patient Preparation and Exposure

Anesthesia and patient preparation are performed per routine TKA protocols. A standard medial parapatellar approach is used, incorporating the previous UKA incision. The quadriceps tendon is split to the apex of the suprapatellar pouch. Four loops of size 0 Vicryl suture are placed at the

apex to prevent tearing into the quadriceps muscle. A standard medial parapatellar approach is used to complete the exposure. The undersurface of the patella is resected to allow visualization with minimal soft tissue exposure.

Femoral Preparation

Overgrown bone is removed from the medial aspect of the femoral component. A drill hole is created in the distal femur for insertion of a standard intramedullary guide rod. A standard TKA distal femoral resection guide then is fixated into position. The femoral prosthesis should not be removed at this time. A standard, thick saw blade is used to resect the distal femur at the 9-mm level. It is important to resect all bone visible around the prosthetic system, taking care to undermine the bone adjacent to the fin of the prosthesis (Fig. 1.10). A small saw blade is used to strip all remaining bone visible around the prosthetic system. A small osteotome then is used to remove the excess bone that has been previously undermined from the initial saw cut.

The femoral prosthesis is 3 mm in thickness and the femoral cutting guide is set at 9 mm; therefore, 5–6 mm of fin and post are exposed by this technique, with the surface of the femoral

Femoral Resection Necessary for Conversion to TKA

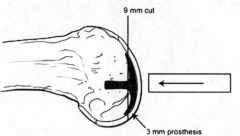

9 mm cut

3 mm prosthesis

Fig. 1.11 Illustration depicting the femoral resection necessary for conversion to TKA in relation to the thickness of the UKA in femoral prosthetic component

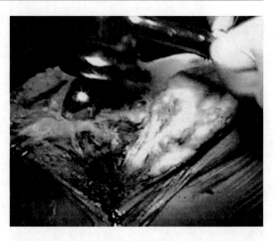

Fig. 1.12 Removal of the UKA femoral prosthetic component, using the post of the prosthesis as a punch and the fin as an osteotome. This technique disrupts the bone-cement interface without damage to the femoral condyles or bone loss

prosthesis sitting 5–6 mm proud of the distal femoral surface cut (Fig. 1.11). The remaining exposed bone is removed from the fin and the posterior aspect of the femoral prosthesis with a small saw blade. The saw is placed posteriorly along the posterior aspect of the femoral condyle to ensure that the bony interface has been properly exposed.

At this time, any attempt to drive the femoral prosthesis off the femur risks the development of a serious fracture or loss of a significant portion of the femoral condyle. The surface of the prosthesis, therefore, is tapped into the distal femur with a hammer. The post of the prosthesis acts as a punch and is driven somewhat into the bone. The fin serves as an osteotome, allowing disruption of the bone-cement interface without damage to the condyles or bone loss (Fig. 1.12). The femoral prosthesis then is grasped and removed from the femoral condyle without bone loss.

Tibial Preparation

The all-polyethylene inlay tibial component is 6.5 mm in thickness. The standard TKA tibial cutting guide is set at 10 mm for 10 mm of resection. It is not necessary to remove the prosthesis. By simply cutting below it,, the medial tibial buttress is preserved, which allows adequate bone support for TKA (Fig. 1.13). This step is performed prior to the final femoral resection to allow adequate space for insertion of the distal femoral resection guide.

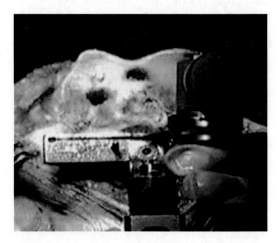

Fig. 1.13 Tibial resection with removal of the UKA tibial prosthetic component

Final Femoral Preparation

The distal femoral resection guide is applied using Whiteside's anteroposterior (AP) axis line as a mid-guide due to the defect in the posterior aspect of the femoral condyle. Standard saw cuts are used to create the necessary distal surfaces. As when performing a standard TKA, it is important to remove the posterior femoral osteophytes.

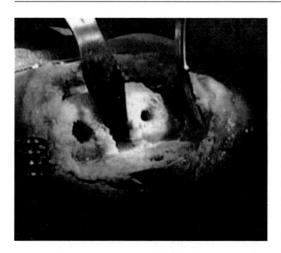

Fig. 1.14 Completion of the femoral and tibial preparations in preparation of insertion of the TKA prosthetic system. Because the UKA prosthetic system has been removed with minimal bone loss, this conversion procedure may be considered delayed primary TKA

At this point, the UKA prosthetic system has been removed with minimal bone loss and the appropriate femoral and tibial preparations are complete (Fig. 1.14). The TKA may proceed with insertion of the desired TKA prosthetic design per standard procedures.

Results

This MIS UKA approach with medial inlay preparation was utilized in a retrospective study comprised of 136 patients classified with Ahlback stages 2, 3, or 4 OA.31 A resurfacing UKA design, the Repicci II unicondylar knee system, was used in all cases. All patients ambulated with a walker within 4 h after surgery and most (98%) were discharged from the hospital within 23 h. The overall revision rate to TKA was 7% at 8 years. Primary TKA designs were used in the eight cases requiring revision, with good (25%) or excellent (75%) Knee Society clinical ratings at follow-up. These results support the safety and efficacy of this MIS UKA technique, illustrate its decreased recovery and rehabilitation time, and substantiate the relative ease of conversion to TKA, if required.

Conclusion

The senior author's multipronged MIS UKA program results in minimal interference in physiology, lifestyle, and future treatment options. The thorough preoperative clinical and radiographic evaluation, which is corroborated by diagnostic arthroscopy, assists in excluding patients with more advanced stages of OA, for whom TKA is the more appropriate treatment choice, thereby reducing morbidity and increasing survivorship of MIS UKA. Because the MIS surgical approach avoids patellar dislocation and nonessential tissue dissection, interference in physiology is averted, which results in lower morbidity and rapid rehabilitation. The resurfacing UKA design diminishes bone resection compared with other UKA designs and, consequently, does not limit future treatment options. Therefore, this MIS UKA may be used in a broader range of patients, including younger, heavier, or more active patients. Combined with the structured pain management program, MIS UKA may be performed on an outpatient basis, with full independence achieved within 4 h postoperatively. The resulting rapid rehabilitation and return to activities of daily living address patient desire to minimize lifestyle interference, thereby enhancing patient satisfaction.

The long-term survivorship of MIS UKA is variable and dependent on many factors, including the state of OA at insertion, the amount of tibial bone support, and material limitations, such as polyethylene deformity and wear. However, because the single most important factor affecting UKA survivorship, regardless of design or use of a MIS approach, is precise surgical technique, proper instructional training is critical in ensuring the surgical expertise required for a successful UKA. Although combining a MIS approach with UKA is appealing, due to lower morbidity and decreased rehabilitation, it adds a significant variable to an already demanding surgical procedure. Proper component positioning and accurate cement removal in the face of decreased visualization is essential. However, once the technique is mastered, this UKA bone-sparing technique combined with the multipronged MIS program is a highly desirable treatment option for patients suffering from unicompartmental OA and has a distinctive role in the orthopedic surgeon's knee prosthetic armamentarium.

References

1. Thornhill TS, Scot RD. Unicompartmental total knee arthroplasty. Orthop Clin North Am 1989;20(2): 245–256
2. Repicci JA, Hartman JF. Minimally invasive unicondylar knee arthroplasty for the treatment of unicompartmental osteoarthritis: an outpatient arthritic bypass procedure. Orthop Clin N Am (2004;35:201–216
3. Repicci JA, Hartman JF. Unicondylar knee replacement: he American experience. In: Fu FH, Browner BD, editors. *Management of osteoarthritis of the knee: an international consensus,* 1st edition. Rosemont, IL: American Academy of Orthopaedic Surgeons, 2003, pp 62–79
4. Repicci JA, Eberle RW. Minimally invasive surgical technique for unicondylar knee arthroplasty. J South Orthop Assoc 1999;8(1):20–27
5. Finthian DC, Kelly MA, Mo VC. Material properties and structure-function relationships in the menisci. Clin Orthop Relat Res 1990 Mar;(252):19–31
6. Grelsamer RP. Current concepts review. Unicompartmental osteorthrosis of the knee. J Bone Joint Surg Am 1995;77(2):278–292
7. Ihn JC, Kim SJ, Park IH. In vitro study of contact area and pressure distribution in the human knee after partial and total meniscectomy. Int Orthop 1993;17(4): 214–218
8. Johnson RJ, Kettelkamp DB, Clark W, et al. Factors affecting late results after meniscectomy. J Bone Joing Surg Am 1974;56(4):719–729
9. Kurosawa H, Fukubayashi T, Nakajima H. Load-bearing mode of the knee joint: physical behavior of the knee joint with or without menisci. Clin Orthop Relat Res 1980 Jun;(149):283–290
10. Shrive NG, O'Connor JJ, Goodfellow JW. Load-bearing in the knee joint. Clin Orthop relat Res 1978 Mar-Apr;(131):279–287
11. Walker PS, Erkman MJ. The role of the menisci in force transmission across the eknee. Clin Orthop Relat Res 1975;(109):84–192
12. Marmour L. Results of single compartment arthroplasty with acrylic cement fixation. A minimum follow-up of two years. Clin Orthop Relat Res 1977 Jan-Feb;(122): 181–188
13. Bohm I, Landsiedl F. Revision surgery after failed nicompartmental knee arthroplasty. A study of 35 cases. J Arthroplasty 2000;15(8):982–989
14. Goodfellow JW, Kershaw CJ, Benson MK et al. The Oxford knee for unicompartmental osteoarthritis. The first 103 cases. J Bone Joint Surg Br 1988;70(5): 692–701
15. Goodfellow JW, Tibrewal SB, Sherman KP, et al. Unicompartmental Oxford meniscal knee arthroplasty. J Arthroplasty 1987;2(1):1–9
16. Kennedy WR, White RP. Unicompartmental arthroplasty of the knee. Postoperative alignment and its influence on overall results. Clin Orthop Relat Ares 1987 Aug;(221):278–285
17. Kozinn SC, Scott R. Unicondylar knee arthroplasty. J Bone Joint Surg Am 1989;71(1):145–150
18. Laskin RS. Unicompartmental tibiofemoral resurfacing arthroplasty. J Bone Joint Surg Am 1978:60(2): 182–185
19. Marmor L. Marmor modular knee in unicompartmental diseases. Minimum four year follow-up. J Bone Joint Surg Am 1979;61(3):347–353
20. Marmor L. Unicompartmental knee arthroplasty. Ten-to 13-year follow-up study. Clin Orthop Relat Res 1988 Jan;(226):14–20
21. Murray DW, Goodfellow JW, O'Connor JJ. The Oxford medial unicompartmental arthroplasty: a ten-year survival study. J Bone Joint Surg Br 1998;80(6): 983–989
22. Squire MW, Callaghan JJ, Goetz DD, et al. Unicompartmental knee replacement. A minimum 15 year follow-up study. Clin Orthop Relat Res 1999 Oct;(367):61–72
23. Stockelman RE, Pohl KP. The long-term efficacy of unicompartmental arthroplasty of the knee. Clin Orthop Relat Res 1991 Oct;(271):88–95
24. Swank M, Stulberg SD, Jiganti J, et al. The natural history of unicompartmental arthroplasty. An eight-year follow-up study with survival analysis. Clin Orthop Relat Res 1993 Jan;(286):130–142
25. Tabor OB, Jr. Tabor OB. Unicompartmental arthroplasty: a long-term follow-up study. J Arthroplasty 1998;13(4):373–379
26. Brown A. The Oxford unicompartmental knee replacement for osteoarthritis. Issues Emerg Health Technol 2001;23:1–4
27. Deshmukh RV, Scott RD. Unicompartmental knee arthroplasty: long-term results. Clin Orthop Relat Res 2001 Nov;(392):272–278
28. Keys GW. Reduced invasive approach for Oxford II medial unicompartmental knee replacement—a preliminary study. Knee 1999; 6(3):193–196
29. Murray DW. Unicompartmental knee replacement: now or never? Orthopedics 2000;23(9):979–980
30. Price A, Webb J, Topf H, et al. Oxford unicompartmental knee replacement with a minimally invasive technique. J Bone Joint Surg Br 2000;82(Suppl 1):24
31. Romanowski MR, Repicci JA. Minimally invasive unicondylar arthroplasty. Eight-year follow-up. Am J Knee Surg 2002;15(1):17–22
32. Price AJ, Webb J, Topf H, Dodd CA, Goodfellow JW, Murray DW. Rapid recovery after Oxford unicompartmental arthroplasty through a short incision. J Arthroplasty 2001;16(8):970–976
33. Brreett WP, Scot RD. Revision of failed unicondylar unicompartmental knee arthroplasty. J Bone Joint Surg Am 1987;69(9):1328–1335

34. Padgett DE, Stern SH, Insall JN. Revision total knee arthroplasty for failed unicompartmental replacement. J Bone Joing Surg Am 1991;73(2):186–90

35. Insall J, Dethmers DA. Revision of total knee arthroplasty. Clin Orthop Relat Res 1982 Oct;(170):123–130

36. Rand JA, Bryan RS. Results of revision total knee arthroplasties using condylar prostheses. A review of fifty knees. J Bone Joing Surg Am 1988;70(5):738–745

37. Kozinn SC, Scott RD. Surgical treatment of unicompartmental degenerative arthritis of the knee. Rheum Dis Clin North Am 1988;14(3):545–564

38. Ahlback S. Osteoarthritis of the knee. A radiographic investigation. Acta Radiol Diagn 1968;277(Suppl): 7–72

39. Romanowski MR, Repicci JA. Unicondylar knee surgery: development of the minimally invasive surgical approach. In: Scuderi GR, Tria AJ, Jr, editor. *MIS of the hip and knee: a clinical perspective.* New York: Springer, 2004. pp 123–151

40. Sisto DJ, Blazina ME, Heskiaoff D, et al. Unicompartmental arthroplasty for osteoarthrosis of the knee. Clin Orthop Relat Res 1993 May;(286):149–153

41. Carr A, Keyes G, Miller R, et al. Medial unicompartmental arthroplasty. A survival study of the Oxford meniscal knee. Clin Orthp Relat Res 1993 Oct;(295): 149–153

42. Jackson RW. Surgical treatment. Osteotomy and unicompartmental arthroplasty. Am J Knee Surg 1998; 11(1):55–57

43. Marmor L. Unicompartmental arthroplasty of the knee with a minimum ten-year follow-up period. Clin Orthop Relat Res 1988 Mar;(228):171–177

44. Cartier P, Sanouiller JL, Grelsamer RP. Unicompartmental knee arthroplasty surgery: 10-year minimum follow-up period. J Arthroplasty 1996; 11(7):782–788

45. Christensen NO. Unicompartmental prosthesis for gonarthrosis. A nine-year series of 575 knees from a Swedish hospital. Clin Orthop Relat Res 1991 Dec;(273):165–169

46. Voss F, Scheinkop MB, Galante JO, et al. Miller-Galante unicompartmental knee arthroplasty at 2- to 5-year follow-up evaluations. J Arthroplasty 1995; 10(6):764–771

47. Berger RA, Nedef DD, Barden RM, et al. Unicompartmental knee arthroplasty. Clinical experience at 6- to 10-year follow-up. Clin Orthop Relat Res 1999 Oct;(367):50–60

48. Bert JM. 10-year survivorship of metal-backed, unicompartmental arthroplasty. J Arthroplasty 1998; 13(8):901–905

49. Capra SW, R., Fehring TK. Unicondylar arthroplasty. A survivorship analysis. J Arthroplasaty 1992; 7(3):247–251

50. Hawker GA, Wright JG, Coyte PC, et al. Determining the need for hip and knee arthroplasty: the role of clinical severity and patients' preferences. Med Care 2001;39:206–216

51. Knutson K, Leold S, Robertsson O, et al. The Swedish knee arthroplasty register. A nation-wide study of 30,003 knees 1976–1992. Acta Orthop Scand 1994;65:375–386

52. Scott RD, Cobb AG, McQueary FG, et al. Unicompartmental knee arthroplasty. Eight- to 12-year follow-up evaluation with survivorship analysis. Clin Orthop Relat Res 1991 Oct;(271):96–100

53. Keblish, PA. The case for unicompartmental knee arthroplasty. Orthopedics 1994;17:853–855

54. Repicci JA, Hartman JF. Minimally invasive surgery for unicondylar knee arthroplasty: the bone-sparing technique. In: Scuderi GR, Tria AJ, Jr, Berger RA, editors. *MIS techniques in orthopedics.* New York: Springer Science + Business Media, Inc., 2006. pp. 193–213

55. Kapandji IA. *The physiology of the joints,* 5th edition, volume 2. New York: Churchill Livingstone, 1987

Minimally Invasive Surgery for Unicondylar Knee Arthroplasty: The Intramedullary Technique*

2

Richard A. Berger and Alfred J. Tria Jr.

Minimally invasive surgery (MIS) for unicondylar knee arthroplasty (UKA) was instituted in the early 1990s by John Repicci [1, 2]. While there had been a long history of UKA dating back to the early 1970s [3–6], the techniques and surgical approaches were modeled after total knee arthroplasty (TKA). The results were not equal to TKA and many surgeons abandoned the procedure. The MIS approach introduced a new method to perform the surgery and helped to improve the results by emphasizing the differences between TKA and UKA. MIS forced the surgeon to consider UKA as a separate operation with its own techniques and its own principles.

*Adapted from Berger RA, Tria AJ, Jr., Minimally invasive surgery for unicondylar knee arthroplasty: the intramedullary technique, in Scuderi GR, Tria, AJ, Jr., Berger RA (eds.), MIS Techniques in Orthopedics, 2006, with kind permission of Springer Science+Business Media.

R.A. Berger (✉)
Department of Orthopaedic Surgery,
Rush-Presbyterian-St. Luke's Medical Center,
Chicago, IL, USA
e-mail: r.a.berger@sbcglobal.net

A.J. Tria Jr.
Department of Orthopaedic Surgery,
UMDNJ-Robert Wood Johnson Hospital,
One Robert Wood Johnson Place, New Brunswick,
NJ, USA

Department of Orthopedic Surgery, Robert Wood
Johnson Medical School, Piscataway, NJ, USA

Preoperative Planning

The preoperative evaluation of the patient should include the history, physical examination, and X-ray. It is critical to choose the correct patient for the operation and to observe the limitations that it imposes. The patient should identify a single compartment of the knee as the primary source of the pain. The physical examination should correlate with the history. Tenderness should be isolated to one tibiofemoral compartment and the patellofemoral exam should be negative. The posterior cruciate and collateral ligaments should be intact with distinct endpoints. The literature suggests that the anterior cruciate ligament (ACL) should be intact [7]; however, the authors will accept some ACL laxity when implanting a fixed bearing UKA. If a mobile bearing device is planned, the ACL should be intact or the knee should have enough anterior to posterior stability to eliminate the need for the ACL. Any existing varus or valgus deformity does not have to be completely correctable to neutral; but the procedure is more difficult to perform with fixed deformity. The range of motion in flexion should be greater than 105°.

The standing X-ray is the primary imaging study (Fig. 2.1). While it is ideal to have a full view of the hip, knee, and ankle, it is not absolutely necessary. The 14×17-in. standard cassette allows measurement of the anatomic axes of the femur and the tibia, which will permit adequate preoperative planning for the surgical procedure.

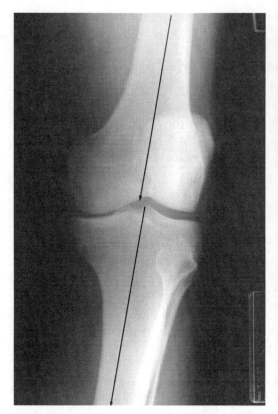

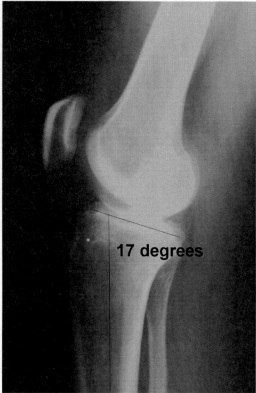

Fig. 2.1 Anteroposterior standing X-ray of a left knee (From Choi YJ, Tanavalee A, Chan A, et al. Unicondylar knee arthroplasty: Surgical approach and early results of the minimally invasive surgical approach, in Scuderi GR, Tria AJ Jr, (eds.), MIS of the Hip and the Knee: A Clinical Perspective. New York, Springer, 2004 with kind permission of Springer Science + Business Media)

Fig. 2.2 Lateral X-ray of the knee showing a 17° tibial slope (From Choi YJ, Tanavalee A, Chan A, et al. Unicondylar knee arthroplasty: Surgical approach and early results of the minimally invasive surgical approach, in Scuderi GR, Tria AJ Jr, (eds.), MIS of the Hip and the Knee: A Clinical Perspective. New York, Springer, 2004, with kind permission of Springer Science + Business Media)

An anteroposterior flexed knee view (notch view) is helpful to rule out any involvement of the opposite condyle. The patellar view, such as a Merchant, will allow evaluation of that area of the knee and will confirm that there is no significant malalignment. The lateral X-ray is used to further judge the patellofemoral joint and to measure the slope of the tibial plateau (Fig. 2.2). The tibial slope can vary from 0 to 15° and can be changed during the surgery to adjust the flexion-extension gap balancing.

The X-rays are important guidelines for the surgery. The varus deformity should not exceed 10°; the valgus should not exceed 15°; and the flexion contracture should not exceed 10°. It is ideal if the varus or valgus deformity corrects to

neutral with passive stress. Deformities outside these limits will require soft tissue releases and corrections that are not compatible with UKA. There should be minimal translocation of the tibia beneath the femur (Fig. 2.3) and the opposite tibiofemoral compartment, and the patellofemoral compartment should show minimal involvement. Translocation indicates that the opposite femoral condyle has degenerative changes and this will certainly compromise the clinical result. While Stern and Insall indicated only 6% of all patients satisfy the requirements for the UKA [8], the authors have found the incidence to be approximately 10–15%. This incidence is, however, decreasing as the minimally invasive TKAs are beginning to flourish. It is best

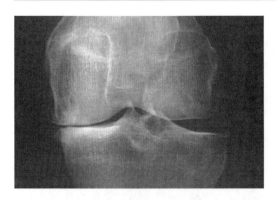

Fig. 2.3 Translocation of the lateral tibial spine contacting the lateral femoral condyle on a standing anteroposterior X-ray of the knee. This is a relative contraindication to UKA (From Choi YJ, Tanavalee A, Chan A, et al. Unicondylar knee arthroplasty: Surgical approach and early results of the minimally invasive surgical approach, in Scuderi GR, Tria AJ Jr, (eds.), MIS of the Hip and the Knee: A Clinical Perspective. New York, Springer, 2004, with kind permission of Springer Science+Business Media)

to observe the strict limitations for the procedure because it will insure a higher rate of success in the cases that are performed.

Magnetic resonance imaging (MRI) is sometimes helpful for evaluation of an avascular necrosis of the femoral condyle or to confirm the integrity of the meniscus in the opposite compartment when the patient complains of an element of instability. However, MRI is not necessary on a routine basis.

Scintigraphic studies are sometimes helpful to identify the extent of involvement of one compartment versus the other. However, once again, this is not a routine diagnostic test.

Surgical Technique (Intramedullary Approach)

The operation can be performed with epidural, spinal, or general anesthesia. Femoral nerve blocks have become very popular but the authors do have some hesitation concerning the technique because of the occasional associated motor block that inhibits the patient's ability to move the knee through active range of motion immediately after the surgical procedure. It is important that the anesthesia team understands that the patients will be required to walk and begin physical therapy within 2–4 h of the completion of the operation and the anesthesia must be in harmony with this approach and with possible discharge to home on the day of the surgical procedure.

The surgery is usually performed with an arterial tourniquet; however, this is not mandatory. The limited MIS incision necessitates continuous repositioning of the knee. The surgeon should be prepared for this and the authors have found that a leg-holding device facilitates the exposure (Fig. 2.4).

The incision is made on either the medial or the lateral side of the patella (depending on the compartment to be replaced) at the superior aspect and is carried distally to the tibial joint line. It is typically 7- to 10-cm long. The incision should not be centered on the joint line because this will limit the exposure to the femoral condyle. In the varus knee, the arthrotomy is performed in a vertical fashion and the authors initially included a short, transverse cut in the capsule approximately 1–2 cm beneath the vastus medialis (Fig. 2.5). The capsular extension is helpful when the surgeon's experience is limited and when exposure is difficult in the "tight" knee. With greater experience, the extension is not necessary. The transverse cut is not a subvastus approach and is an incision in the capsule of the knee midway between the vastus medialis and the tibial joint line. The deep MCL is released on the tibial side to improve the exposure of the joint. The release is not performed for the purposes of alignment correction. This is the beginning of the divergence of the UKA from the TKA surgery. It is important to remember that the surgery is only performed on one side of the joint. The goal of the surgery is to replace one side and to balance the forces so that the arthroplasty and the opposite compartment share the weight bearing equally. If the medial ligamentous complex is released, there is the potential for overloading the opposite side, with resultant pain and failure.

In the lateral UKA, the "T" extension is not necessary. The vertical incision is taken down to the tibial plateau and the iliotibial band (ITB) is sharply released from Gerdy's tubercle and elevated posteriorly (Fig. 2.6). The arthrotomy is

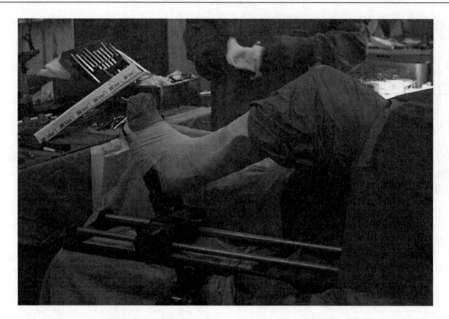

Fig. 2.4 The leg holder (Innovative Medical Products, Inc., Plainville, Connecticut) allows flexion and extension of the knee along with internal and external rotation (From Choi YJ, Tanavalee A, Chan A, et al. Unicondylar knee arthroplasty: Surgical approach and early results of the minimally invasive surgical approach, in Scuderi GR, Tria AJ Jr, (eds.), MIS of the Hip and the Knee: A Clinical Perspective. New York, Springer, 2004, with kind permission of Springer Science + Business Media)

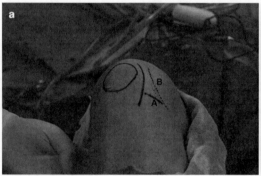
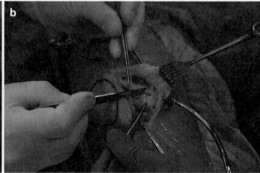

Fig. 2.5 (a) The medial incision extends from the top of the patella to just below the tibial joint line (*A*). *B* is the outline of the margin of the medial femoral condyle. (b) The medial arthrotomy can include a "T" in the capsule (made with the tip of the knife blade) (From Scuderi GR, Tria AJ Jr, MIS of the Hip and the Knee: A Clinical Perspective. New York, Springer, 2004, with kind permission of Springer Science + Business Media.)

closed in a vertical fashion and the ITB is left to scar down to the tibial metaphysis.

The patella is not everted in the procedure and the vastus medialis is not violated either by a dividing incision or a subvastus approach. The sparing of the surrounding soft tissue structures and the preservation of the extensor mechanism in its entirety makes the procedure minimally invasive.

With the completion of the arthrotomy, the peripheral osteophytes should be removed from the femoral condyle and the tibial plateau. All compartments of the joint should be inspected. It is not unusual to see some limited arthritic involvement in the other compartments of the knee. The preoperative evaluation should be thorough enough to preclude a conversion to a TKA. Diagnostic arthroscopy is not necessary

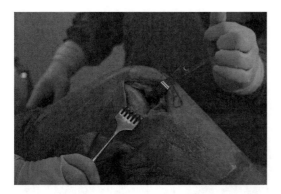

Fig. 2.6 The lateral view of a right knee shows the anterior tibial joint line after the iliotibial band has been released and retracted posteriorly (From Choi YJ, Tanavalee A, Chan A, et al. Unicondylar knee arthroplasty: Surgical approach and early results of the minimally invasive surgical approach, in Scuderi GR, Tria AJ Jr, (eds.), MIS of the Hip and the Knee: A Clinical Perspective. New York, Springer, 2004, with kind permission of Springer Science + Business Media)

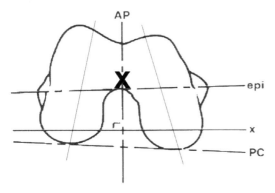

Fig. 2.7 The intramedullary hole is located just above the roof of the intercondylar notch (marked with the letter "*X*") (Adapted from Choi YJ, Tanavalee A, Chan A, et al. Unicondylar knee arthroplasty: Surgical approach and early results of the minimally invasive surgical approach, in Scuderi GR, Tria AJ Jr, (eds.), MIS of the Hip and the Knee: A Clinical Perspective. New York, Springer, 2004, with kind permission of Springer Science + Business Media)

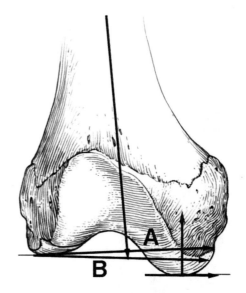

Fig. 2.8 The two cuts on the medial femoral condyle show that the deeper resection (line "*A*") results in less valgus than line "*B*" (3° versus 5°). This also allows for more space in full extension (From Tria AJ, Klein KS. An Illustrated Guide to the Knee. New York, Churchill Livingstone, 1992, with permission of Elsevier, Inc.)

but can sometimes be included to confirm the anatomy of the opposite side in an unusual case. The addition of this procedure should be undertaken with care to avoid the possibility of increasing the associated infection rate.

The intramedullary technique requires an entrance hole centered just above the roof of the intercondylar notch (Fig. 2.7). The intramedullary canal is suctioned free of its contents to decrease fat embolization and the instrument is set into the canal.

The depth of the distal femoral cut affects the extension gap and also the anatomic valgus of the distal femur (Fig. 2.8). The angle (or tilt) of the cut determines the perpendicularity of the component to the tibial plateau surface in full extension (Fig. 2.9). This angle can be precisely determined by measuring the difference between the anatomic and mechanical axis of the knee on long standing X-ray films. In the clinical setting, the authors arbitrarily choose a 4° angle for the varus knee and a 6° angle for the valgus knee.

Flexion contractures of the knee can be corrected with the medial UKA but not with the lateral replacement. If there is a flexion contracture and the distal anatomic femoral valgus is 5° or less in the varus knee, the standard amount of bone is removed to be replaced millimeter for millimeter with the prosthesis. If the distal femoral valgus is 6° or more in the varus knee, 2 mm of additional bone is removed from the distal femur to decrease the excess valgus and to increase the space in full extension. Increasing the space in full extension helps to correct the flexion contracture and enables the surgeon to decrease the associated depth of the tibial cut.

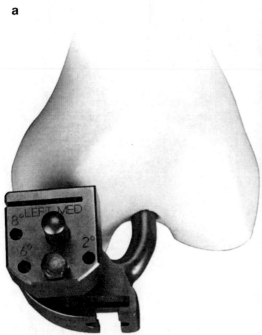

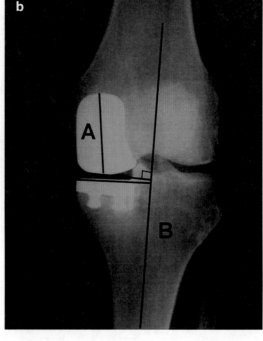

Fig. 2.9 (**a**) The intramedullary guide allows for a distal cut of 2, 4, 6, or 8°. This setting adjusts the angle of the femoral component with relation to the tibial plateau cut surface. It does not adjust the overall varus or valgus of the knee because it is only cutting one condyle. (**b**) The femoral comvponent "tilt" is defined as the angle between the long axis of the component (line "*A*") referenced to the axis of the tibial shaft (line "*B*"). (**a**, From Berger RA, Tria AJ Jr, Minimally invasive surgery for unicondylar knee arthroplasty: the intramedullary technique, in Scuderi GR, Tria AJ Jr, Berger RA (eds.), MIS Techniques in Orthopedics, 2006, with kind permission of Springer Science+Business Media)

The deeper femoral cut saves 2 mm of bone on the tibial side and results in a total distal femoral resection of 8 mm. The resection does not elevate the femoral joint line as it would in a TKA. Most TKA femoral components remove a minimum of 9 mm for the prosthesis so that this change does not adversely affect revision to a TKA.

In the valgus knee, the maximum acceptable deformity is 15° and the distal femur is cut millimeter for millimeter for replacement. The deformity will be slightly decreased with a standard resurfacing because the prosthesis and the cement mantle are slightly thicker than the bone that is removed. Because the lateral femoral condyle is less prominent than the medial condyle in full extension, flexion contractures cannot be corrected as easily on the lateral side. A deeper cut on the lateral femoral condyle will only increase the distal femoral valgus without changing the extension gap significantly.

After completing the distal femoral cut, it is easier to proceed to the tibial preparation because this in turn opens up the space in 90° of flexion and makes the femoral finishing cuts much easier. The tibial cut is made with an extramedullary instrument (Fig. 2.10). In the MIS setting, intramedullary instrumentation is difficult on the tibial side without everting the patella. The tibial cut can be angled from anterior to posterior. Most systems favor a 5–7° posterior slope for roll back. The slope of the cut also affects the flexion–extension balancing. The balancing is not the same as the techniques for TKA. In the UKA surgery, the flexion gap is usually larger than the extension gap because of the flexion contracture that is present in almost all arthritic knees. As the flexion contracture increases to 10°, the extension gap becomes tighter. If the slope of the tibial cut is decreased from the anatomic slope of the preoperative tibial X-ray, the cut can be made deeper anteriorly to give greater space in extension while maintaining the same flexion gap posteriorly (Fig. 2.11). This is the alternate technique for flexion contracture correction if the distal femoral valgus is normal at 5° or less.

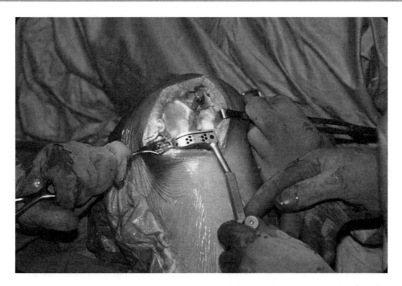

Fig. 2.10 The tibial cut is complete with an extramedullary guide (From Berger RA, Tria AJ Jr, Minimally invasive surgery for unicondylar knee arthroplasty: the intramedullary technique, in Scuderi GR, Tria AJ Jr, Berger RA (eds.), MIS Techniques in Orthopedics, 2006, with kind permission of Springer Science + Business Media)

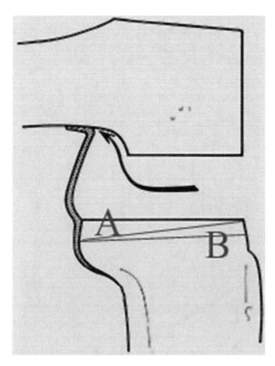

Fig. 2.11 The slope of the tibial cut can be changed to correct flexion-extension imbalance. The flexion gap is often larger than the extension gap. The cut "*A*" can be lowered anteriorly and the slope decreased to line "*B*," which will equalize the gaps. (From Berger RA, Tria AJ Jr, Minimally invasive surgery for unicondylar knee arthroplasty: the intramedullary technique, in Scuderi GR, Tria AJ Jr, Berger RA (eds.), MIS Techniques in Orthopedics, 2006, with kind permission of Springer Science + Business Media)

With the completion of the tibial cut, the remainder of the femoral cuts can be completed with the appropriate blocks for guidance of the saws. An intramedullary retractor can be used to retract the patella (Fig. 2.12). The femoral runner should be a slight bit smaller than the original femoral condyle surface and it should be perpendicular to the tibial plateau at 90° of flexion and centered medial to lateral on the condyle. If the femoral condyle divergence is extreme in 90° of flexion, the femoral component should be positioned perpendicular to the tibial cut surface (parallel to the long axis of the tibia). This positioning may result in some overhang of the femoral runner into the intercondylar notch (Fig. 2.13).

The tibial tray should cover the entire cut surface out to the cortical rim without overhang on the medial or lateral side of the tibia. The component is not inlayed and any degree of varus positioning should be avoided. The inlay technique depends upon the subchondral bone surface for support and if this is violated during the tibial preparation, sinkage of the component will certainly follow. Varus inclination can lead to early component loosening and should be avoided.

Once the cuts are completed, the flexion–extension gap should be tested with the trial components in position. In the ideal case, there should be 2 mm of laxity in both positions (Fig. 2.14). It is best not to over tighten the joint and to accept greater rather than less laxity. Excess tightness may lead to early polyethylene failure and also contributes to increase pressure transmission to the opposite side.

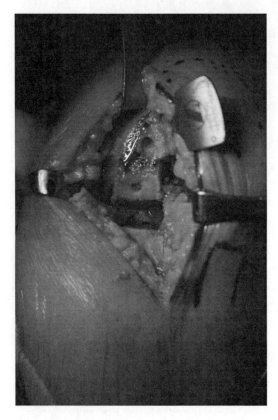

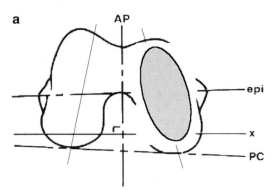

Fig. 2.12 The intramedullary retractor is useful to visualize the joint (labeled with "Z")

Three separate items determine the overall varus or valgus of the knee: the depth of the tibial cut, the tibial polyethylene thickness, and the depth of the femoral cut. The tibia can be cut exactly perpendicular and the distal femoral cut can be set in 4° of valgus; but with the insertion of an excessively thick polyethylene, the knee can be shifted into 6 or more degrees of valgus and overcorrected despite properly aligned bone cuts. In the setting of the TKA, changing the thickness of the tibial insert affects spacing in full extension and 90° of flexion but it does not affect the varus or valgus of the knee, which remain the same.

If the UKA spacing is not symmetric, the tibial cut should be altered. Typically, the extension space will be smaller than the flexion space. This can be corrected by starting the tibial cut slightly deeper on the anterior surface and decreasing the slope angle. Once again, in TKA, the extension space is easily increased by removing more bone from the distal femur. In UKA, deepening the femoral cut will change the distal femoral valgus and will also increase the size of the component because the anteroposterior surface will be increased. This may lead to poor bone contact with the new femoral component and possible early loosening. Thus, it is best to modify the spacing with changes on the tibial side. If the space in extension is larger than the flexion space, this usually means that the slope of the tibial cut was made too shallow and the slope should just be increased.

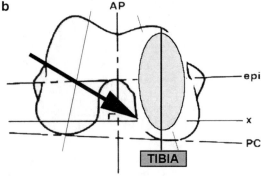

Fig. 2.13 (**a**) If the femoral component is aligned with the cut articular surface of the femur, the divergence of the condyles may be too great and the subsequent position may lead to edge loading on the polyethylene tibial insert.

(**b**) The femoral component should be perpendicular to the tibial insert even if this leads to a non-anatomic position on the femoral surface and slight overhang of the component into the intercondylar notch

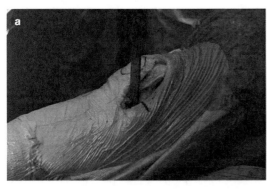
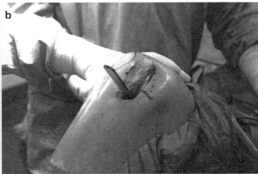

Fig. 2.14 (**a**) The tongue depressor is 2-mm thick and demonstrates the proper laxity in full extension of the knee. (**b**) The tongue depressor demonstrates the matching proper laxity in 90° of flexion (From Choi YJ, Tanavalee A, Chan A, et al. Unicondylar knee arthroplasty: Surgical approach and early results of the minimally invasive surgical approach, in Scuderi GR, Tria AJ Jr, (eds.), MIS of the Hip and the Knee: A Clinical Perspective. New York, Springer, 2004, with kind permission of Springer Science + Business Media)

After testing the components for stability, range of motion, and flexion–extension balance, the final components are cemented in place. Cementless fixation for UKA has not been very successful and the authors do not recommend that approach. When the tibial component is a modular design, the metal tray can be cemented in place first and this allows excellent visualization of the posterior aspect of the joint and also allows more space for the femoral component cementing. The all-polyethylene insert does give more thickness to the prosthesis. However, the thicker polyethylene blocks visualization for the cementing; and, if full thickness polyethylene failure occurs, the exchange will require invasion of the underlying tibial bone. The modular tibial tray allows polyethylene exchange without bone invasion and backside wear is not a problem in UKA surgery. The femoral runner is cemented after the tibial tray, and the polyethylene is inserted last.

The tourniquet is released before the closure and adequate hemostasis is established. The closure is completed in the standard technique with special attention to be sure that the vastus medialis is well reattached to the patella to allow early and rapid range of motion of the knee.

At the time of the closure, the posterior capsule and the surrounding structures can be infiltrated with anesthetic agents to help with the early postoperative physical therapy.

Results

At present there are few reports using the MIS surgical approach. Berger's report [9] included a 10-year follow-up with 98% longevity using standard open arthrotomy techniques. The average age of the patients was 68 years old and the indications for the procedure were quite strict. His second report extended the follow up to 13 years with a survival rate of 95.7% [10]. Price reported early follow-up of an abbreviated incision for UKA with good results [11]. He compared 40 Oxford UKAs using an MIS-type incision with 20 Oxford UKAs performed with a standard incision. The average rate of recovery of the MIS UKAs was twice as fast. The accuracy of the implantation was evaluated using 11 variables on fluoroscopically centered postoperative X-rays and was found to be the same as the open UKAs. Price concluded that more rapid recovery was possible with less morbidity. The technique did not compromise the final result of the UKA. Repicci reported on 136 knees with 8 years of follow-up using the MIS technique [2]. There were ten revisions (7%): three for technical errors, one for poor pain relief, five for advancing disease, and one for fracture. The revisions for technical errors occurred from 6 to 25 months after surgery. The revisions for advancing disease occurred from 37 to 90 months after surgery.

Repicci concluded that MIS UKA is "... an initial arthroplasty procedure (that) relieves pain, restores limb alignment, and improves function with minimal morbidity without interfering with future TKA."

The senior author has performed 385 UKAs using the Miller-Galante Unicondylar Knee Arthroplasty (Zimmer, Warsaw, IN). Fifty-seven patients underwent UKA in the first year (2000). Forty-one (72%) patients have 2 or more years of follow up [12]. There were 24 women and 17 men, including six bilateral surgeries, four simultaneous, and two staged 6–8 weeks apart. There were 47 knees, 45 varus and 2 valgus. The average age was 68 years old, with a range from 42 to 93 years. Ten patients (30%) were younger than age 60 years and eight patients (20%) were older than age 75 years. The average weight was 189 pounds. The range of motion went from 120° before the operation to 132° after the surgery. One knee was converted to a TKA because of patellar subluxation occurring 9 months after the surgery. The revision was performed at 14 months after the original TKA. One knee was revised to a TKA 5 years after the original surgery because of increasing patellofemoral arthritis. One patient sustained an undisplaced tibial plateau fracture 2 weeks after surgery and this healed without intervention. All patients obtained their full range of motion within 3 weeks. The overall revision rate is 2 (4%) of 47 knees at 6 years after surgery.

In the entire group of 385 UKAs that have been performed since 2000, there have been seven revisions. Five of these revisions were for advancing patellofemoral arthritis, one was for the patellar subluxation mentioned previously, and one was for a femoral component loosening. The femoral component failed because it was too large and impinged upon the patellofemoral joint. While these are very early results, most of the series with poor results started to see the failures within the first 2–5 years following the procedure.

Conclusions

The results of UKA have improved steadily since the late 1990s. The MIS technique has fostered better results and has helped to set UKA apart from TKA in the minds of the operating surgeons. The intramedullary instrumentation has been well adapted to the MIS technique. As the prosthetic designs and surgical techniques continue to improve, MIS UKA should have results similar to those of TKA in the first 10–15 years and give patients a choice before TKA that will permit greater activity and improved quality of life without compromising the result of a later TKA.

References

1. Repicci JA, Eberle RW. Minimally invasive surgical technique for unicondylar knee arthroplasty. J South Orthop Assoc 8(1):20–27, 1999
2. Romanowski MR, Repicci JA. Minimally invasive unicondylar arthroplasty, eight year follow-up. J Knee Surg 15(1):17–22, 2002
3. Marmor L. Marmor modular knee in unicompartmental disease. Minimum four-year follow-up. J Bone Joint Surg Am 61 A(3):347–353, 1979
4. Insall J, Walker P. Unicondylar knee replacement. Clin Orthop Relat Res ; (120):83–85, 1976 Oct
5. Laskin RS Unicompartment tibiofemoral resurfacing arthroplasty. J Bone Joint Surg Am 60A:182–185, 1978
6. Goodfellow J, O'connor J. The mechanics of the knee and prosthesis design. J Bone Joint Surg Br 60B:358–369, 1978
7. Goodfellow JW, Kershaw CJ, Benson MK, O'Connor JJ. The Oxford knee for unicompartmental osteoarthritis. The first 103 cases. J Bone Joint Surg Br 70:692–701, 1988
8. Stern SH, Becker MW, Insall J. Unicompartmental knee arthroplasty. An evaluation of selection criteria. Clin Orthop Relat Res 286:143–148, 1993
9. Berger RA, Nedeff DD, Barden RN, Sheinkop MN, Jacobs JJ, Rosenberg AG, Galante JO. Unicompartmental knee arthroplasty. Clin Orthop Relat Res 367:50–60, 1999
10. Berger RA, Meneghini RM, Jacobs JJ, Sheinkop MB, Della Valle CJ, Rosenberg AG, Galante JO. Results of unicompartmental knee arthroplasty at a minimum of ten years of follow-up. J Bone Joint Surg Am 87:999–1006, 2005
11. Price AJ, Webb J, Topf H, Dodd CAF, Goodfellow JW, Murray DW, Oxford Hip and Knee Group. Rapid recovery after Oxford unicompartmental arthroplasty through a short incision. J Arthroplasty 16:970–976, 2001
12. Gesell MW, Tria AJ, Jr. MIS unicondylar knee arthroplasty: surgical approach and early results. Clin Orthop Relat Res 428:53–60, 2004
13. Choi YJ, Tanavalee A, Chan A, et al. Unicondylar knee arthroplasty: Surgical approach and early results of the minimally invasive surgical approach, in Scuderi GR, Tria AJ Jr, (eds.), MIS of the Hip and the Knee: A Clinical Perspective. New York, Springer, 2004

The Extramedullary Tensor Technique for Unicondylar Knee Arthroplasty*

3

Paul L. Saenger

The extramedullary (EM) tensor tools and surgical technique were developed to orient cutting guides for the implantation of the M/G unicompartmental prosthesis with greater ease and accuracy and to reduce the surgical morbidity of this limited reconstruction. Unicompartmental knee replacement attempts to reduce pain and improve function by restoring the extremity's alignment and the joint's soft tissue balance with the positioning of an implant limited to that compartment. All unicompartmental implants, be they monoblock wafers, mobile bearing devices, or fixed articular prostheses, must effect this restoration to enjoy whatever success they may provide.

Various surgical techniques for their implantation are available. Instrument systems without direct linkage of the femoral and tibial cuts require intuitive estimates. With such a technique, the implant must, in effect, be retrofitted. The cuts are made and then a device of a given volume and width is chosen that best fits the flexion and extension gaps created. Those cuts were not predetermined for a given implant and thus are approximations. Approximations can work well should there be unlimited prosthetic sizes from which to choose.

*Adapted from Saenger PL, Minimally invasive surgery for unicondylar knee arthroplasy: The extramedullary approach, in Scuderi GR, Tria AJ, Berger RA (eds.), MIS Techniques in Orthopedics, 2006, with kind permission of Springer Science + Business Media.

P.L. Saenger (✉)
Private Practice, Blue Ridge Bone & Joint Clinic, PA,
Asheville, NC, USA
e-mail: kcherry@brbj.com

The relationship between the bone cuts and the subsequent insertion of an implant with its particular geometry filling the created extension and flexion gaps, it should be remembered, is the key to the angular and soft tissue balance one is attempting to achieve. Instruments now exist that allow the anticipated cuts to be positioned relative to a knee's corrected posture. There is a direct relationship such that the cuts made are specific for a given implant's dimensions. The EM tensor technique herein described uses patented instrumentation with direct linkage, referencing off the femur and tibia simultaneously. Knowing the dimensions of the intended implant in both extension and flexion allows then the use of cutting guides that create spatial dimensions, that is, extension and flexion gaps, to accommodate a particular composite implant.

The Tensor

The tensor device is an adjustable interposed spacer with incorporated tibial and femoral cutting surfaces that is positioned in extension between the femur and tibia while their articular surfaces are held in a corrected position. The space to be created for a given implant can then be made with a specific width and slope oriented at will prior to setting the surface cutting guides. The relationship of the two cut surfaces is set with respect to a pre-achieved correction of the soft tissue tension and overall limb alignment (Fig. 3.1).

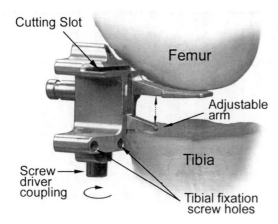

Fig. 3.1 The tensor device

Predetermined flexion and extension gaps lesson the need to modify or compensate for an imbalance potentially created by guesswork. The need for subsequent *eyeball* revisions is reduced. Alignment instruments that measure first and cut second attempt to eliminate the inaccuracies and secondary complexities of the bone preparation.

Minimally Invasive Surgery

Central to developing the EM tensor system was the desire to lessen the morbidity associated with this limited reconstruction. The invasiveness of any surgical procedure is certainly more than the length or the incision. In the case of knee reconstruction, the extent of the quadriceps division, the intrusion of the intramedullary canal [1, 2], or the use of a tourniquet add to the morbidity of the effort. To avoid or limit such compromising elements is the goal of MIS. The tensor technique requires a small skin incision, usually 4–7 cm, a modest division of the vastus medialis oblique (VMO), no intrusion of the intramedullary canal, and there is no need for a tourniquet.

The instruments and implants detailed in this chapter will likely be soon replaced with new versions. However, the concept and use of artificial implants that adhere to the host bone so as to anatomically reconstruct articular surfaces will likely endure. Their surgical implantation will require an ever more accurate and less morbid technique. Understanding the nature of this

implant, the Zimmer M/G unicompartmental, and its attendant EM tensioning instrumentation and technique is apropos to the consideration of future developments.

The Implant

Unicompartmental knee reconstruction using femoral and tibial implants that mimic the original geometry of the host articular surfaces and that are secured to cut bone with cement has been shown to offer reliably good to excellent results [3–8]. Several series have demonstrated the M/G unicompartmental (Zimmer, Inc., Warsaw, IN) prosthesis to offer success for at least 10 years equal to or better than total knee arthroplasty (TKA) in middle aged or older populations [9–11]. The prosthesis consists of a biconvex chrome cobalt femoral component with three precoated backside facets. It is cemented to three matching cut femoral bone surfaces; planed cuts that determined the implant's position and orientation. The tibial implant, either monoblock or modular, is available in incremental widths of 8, 10, 12, and 14 mm. It, too, is cemented to a cut, planed surface (Fig. 3.2).

Measure First, Cut Second

Regardless of future navigational aids for yet-to-be-designed implants, the procedure will likely require orienting the bone preparation for a given implant relative to a specifically corrected and thereafter maintained joint and limb posture.

The tensor technique uses a space-filling tensioner that serves as an adjustable expansive unit between the femur and tibia that maintains the corrected alignment and tissue balance in extension. With that done, the femoral and tibial cutting blocks, using shared fixation screws, are set so as to create a space equal to the intended implant's composite width. The orientation of the surfaces to be cut can be accurately established. As presently configured, those surfaces are parallel to one another in the coronal plane. In the sagittal plane, the slope on the tibia is adjustable to 3°, 5°, or 7°. These cut surface relationships could be readily altered if it is determined to be otherwise optimal (Fig. 3.3a, b).

How Much Correction?

Occasionally, unicompartmental pathology does not involve significant deformity of the joint space and thus the alignment and tissue balance is intact.

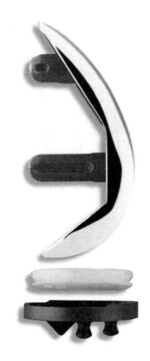

Fig. 3.2 The M/G unicompartmental prosthesis

In that case, maintaining the existing dynamic geometric relationships is a fundamental goal of the procedure. More often, with the eccentric loss of articular and meniscal cartilage seen in unicompartmental disease, the knee falls into varus or valgus. This intraarticular loss secondarily affects the ligamentous stability. By restoring the intraarticular spacing, the ligaments are again tensioned. Assuming there is no soft tissue contracture, replacing the lost cartilage and bone with an implant of equal dimensions should restore both the joint's soft tissue tension and overall alignment relative to the mechanical and anatomical axes.

Alignment and soft tissue balance are critical to the success of TKAs, too. However, it must be understood that the alignment of the extremity as a whole in TKA is a function of the angle of the cuts. That is not true for unicondylar knee arthroplasty (UKA). For instance, in TKA, a 6° femoral cut combined with a standard 0° cut on the tibia can be expected to result in a femoral-tibial angle of 6°. Varying the thickness of the plastic insert will affect the soft tissue tension but not the angle of the extremity's alignment.

Varying the thickness of the insert in a UKA directly affects the soft tissue tension as well. But, unlike the TKA, in a UKA it is an eccentric variation and changes the alignment, too. In that sense, it is similar to the angular alteration seen with wedge resection or insertion used in high tibial osteotomies (HTO). However, unlike HTO, a unicompartmental insert is intraarticular and

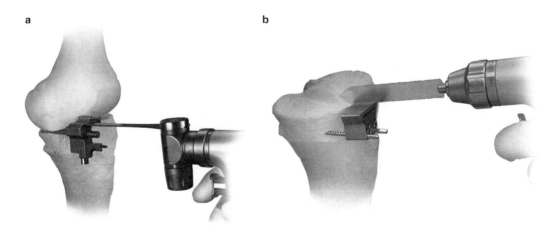

Fig. 3.3 (a) The tensor serves as the distal femoral cutting block held with tibial fixation screws that then (b) support and orient the tibial cutting block

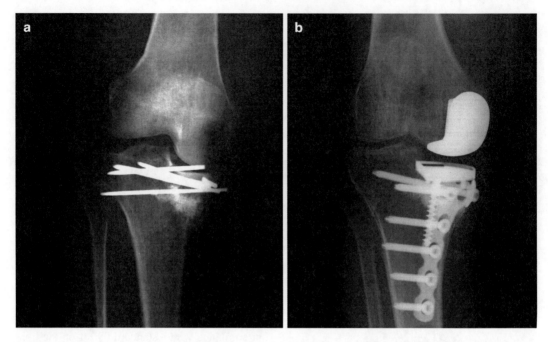

Fig. 3.4 (a) Nonunion with varus 9 months after inadequate fixation of a medial tibial plateau fracture in a 51-year-old woman. (b) Four-year postoperative X-ray of a unicompartmental reconstruction with soft tissue release for a contracture using a Sulzer Natural Knee Uni. Preoperative range of motion (*ROM*), 5–65°; postoperative ROM, 3–122°

thus the addition of a thicker implant will, once the soft tissues are already snug, *overstuff* the joint. Too wide a prosthesis creates intraarticular compressive forces detrimental to not only the implant, but to the uninvolved compartment as well and can be expected to be deleterious to both [12]. It is very important to avoid *overstuffing* the joint throughout its arc of movement from extension to flexion.

The mechanical axis of the lower extremity is that line that passes through the center of the hip, knee, and ankle. This system assumes that a mechanical axis of 0° is a reference point, not a target. It is thought that knees that fall into varus for want of medial cartilage were likely in some varus relative to a 0° mechanical axis even before the pathology notably altered the alignment. Thus, to force that knee to 0° would presumably go beyond what was once normal and in so doing would tighten the medial ligaments beyond their norm. Therefore, when using the mechanical axis as a guide, the correction will typically fall slightly short of full correction to 0° [13].

While the two, alignment and soft tissue tension, are directly related and can each be used to help assess the correction, it is the latter, the soft tissue tension, that is thought to be most critical. Until such time as a more sophisticated method of measuring intracompartmental pressure is used, the present system relies on the manual and visual perceptions of the surgeon such that a valgus stress (or varus in the case of lateral reconstruction) should allow approximately 2 mm of opening. Regardless of the alignment, if the ligaments are too tight and the knee *overstuffed*, the long-term success of the procedure is likely to be compromised.

In the author's experience, most knees thought to be appropriate for this procedure can be adequately corrected without soft tissue release. Indeed, for many knees, there may be little or no angular or ligamentous deformity. However, in selected cases, a correction toward an improved alignment and appropriate soft tissue tension requires the release of the soft tissue contracture (Fig. 3.4a, b).

Surgical Technique

Medial unicompartmental degenerative joint disease can be seen as a disease of extension [14]. Cartilage loss on the femur, for instance, is often minimal on the posterior condyle where it articulates with the tibia in flexion. Rather, the more profound compromise occurs on the distal end of the condyle in the area that articulates with the tibia as the knee extends. Genu varum is an extension deformity. The correction to be made is in extension (Fig. 3.5).

Keying off the distal femur with a cutting guide that allows the reestablishment of the appropriate joint line, the EM tensor, a variable spacing block inserted into the involved compartment, is adjusted to maintain a corrected extension alignment. Secured to both femur and tibia by shared fixation posts, coordinated cutting blocks serve to allow the distal femoral and then the tibial cuts to be made in a directly linked fashion that will prepare this predetermined space to be filled by an anticipated implant (Fig. 3.6a–e).

With the extension pathology restructured, it is time to balance the flexion gap. It is important that the knee not be compromised in flexion by overtensioning or undertensioning the flexion gap with inappropriate bone preparation or inaccurate femoral sizing. To avoid that complication, a gauge is used to predict the ensuing flexion gap. This ensures that the subsequent cut on the posterior femur combined with the cut already made on the tibia creates a flexion space whose soft tissue tension is consistent with that established for extension.

The EM tensor technique is intended to follow sequential steps. Altering the sequence may compromise the end result. With experience, the procedure can be regularly accomplished with a 4–7-cm skin incision, the extent of which has the potential to shrink further with future innovation.

Given the restricted space, the intact ligaments, and the modest incision, adequate exposure requires that the limb be postured and manipulated in specific ways to facilitate the various steps. For instance, knee extension relaxes the quad mechanism and allows displacement of the patella not possible with even slight flexion with the VMO intact. Thus, certain steps are best done in full extension whereas other steps require flexion to as much as 120°. In that case, maintaining a valgus stress while holding the leg externally rotated for a medial reconstruction will, along with the wise use of retractors, enhance greatly the exposure.

The following description of the surgical technique reflects one surgeon's way of doing things. It represents a considered effort to minimize the morbidity and ensure proper implant positioning. It involves obtaining a preoperative anteroposterior (AP) hip X-ray with markers over the hip joint in an effort to determine accurately the mechanical axis as a reference point for limb alignment. Also, the use of a tourniquet is thought to be unnecessary. That unicompartmental procedures are routinely done successfully without X-rays and with tourniquets is recognized. It is also known that large numbers of prosthetic devices of this and similar design have been implanted with reported good results using indirectly linked cutting or measuring guides. That is a credit to the skill and understanding of those surgeons implanting

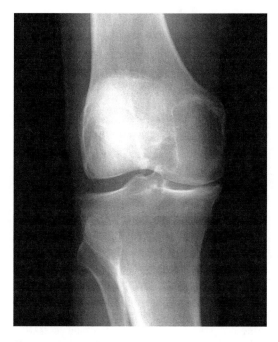

Fig. 3.5 X-ray of medial degenerative joint disease (*DJD*) with varus deformity

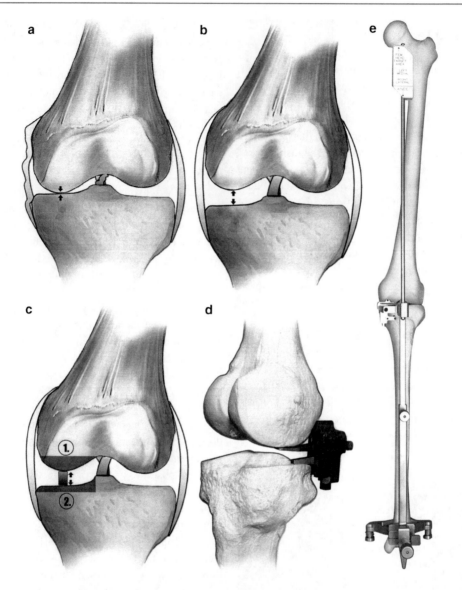

Fig. 3.6 (**a**) The narrowed medial compartment is opened until (**b**) the medial ligaments are tensioned. (**c**) The space is filled with the tensor. (**d**) Setting parallel cuts (1 and 2) for the intended implant. (**e**) Attached alignment rods confirm orientation

the prosthesis. It also suggests the potential and adaptability of these secured implants. The EM tensor technique was developed to lessen the guesswork by providing accurate, reproducible cuts with minimally invasive instruments that can diminish many of the complexities inherent to this procedure.

The great majority of unicompartmental reconstructions are done medially and, of those, most are in middle-aged to older men and women with a narrowed medial compartment secondary to osteoarthritis as seen on physical examination and standing X-rays. The procedure is thus described for that compartment with that pathology in mind and assumes some varus misalignment with associated medial ligament laxity that allows correction without soft tissue release. The steps of the procedure are the same whether this deformity is a little or a lot. Lateral reconstruction is essentially the same other than the incision is made lateral to the patella.

Table 3.1 Surgical steps for extramedullary tensor technique for unicondylar knee arthroplasty

1. Incision
2. Removal of the anterior boss of the tibia
3. Alignment correction
4. Distal femoral cut
5. Tibial cuts
6. Flexion and extension gaps
7. Anterior femoral marking
8. Femoral finishing guide sizing and positioning
9. Tibial sizing and finishing
10. Testing and cementing

Surgical Steps

Incision

The length and position of the incision is dependent on the exposure required for certain surgical steps done in flexion (Table 3.1). In extension, the arthrotomy is a window that can be moved about for better viewing. In flexion, however, the quad is tight and the patella locked into the trochlea. Knowing what must be seen in flexion, that is, the anterior aspect of the distal femur down to the tibial joint line just medial to the patellar tendon, can then serve to guide the proximal and distal extent of the skin and retinaculum incision.

Therefore, with the knee flexed, an incision is made slightly medial to the midline from near the superior pole of the patella to just a few millimeters below the joint line. Likewise, divide the medial retinaculum and fat pad. Excise a portion of the fat pad in the area along with the anterior third of the meniscus. Use electrocautery for hemostasis. Excise osteophytes found on the femur, tibia, and patella. For exposure now and whenever the knee is flexed, use a 90° bent sharp Hohmann retractor positioned in the notch and a similar retractor or two along the medial tibia. Importantly, this also protects the cruciates and medial collateral ligament (MCL) while using saw blades (Figs. 3.7 and 3.8).

Removal of the Anterior Boss of the Tibia

Positioning and manipulating the tensor is made easier by removing the anterior tibial boss normally encountered. With the reciprocating saw,

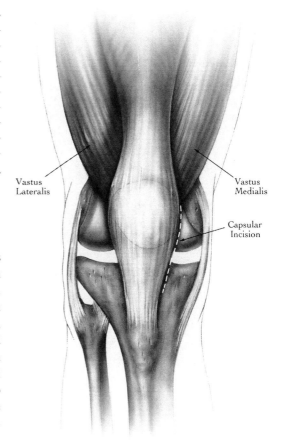

Fig. 3.7 The incision

make a 2- or 3-mm-deep cut along the medial edge of the tibial spine parallel to the tibial axis. Then, with the oscillating saw, remove the tibial boss perpendicular to the tibial axis to a depth of approximately 3 mm. This additional space makes easier the insertion of the spacer arms and also improves the interface between the active (it moves) tibial arm and the surface of the anterior tibial plateau (Fig. 3.9).

Alignment Correction

The tensor and alignment rods are positioned with the knee in extension. To ease their assembly, put the tensor into the joint with the connecting tower attached. Clamp the tibial alignment rod to the distal leg with the locking screws loose

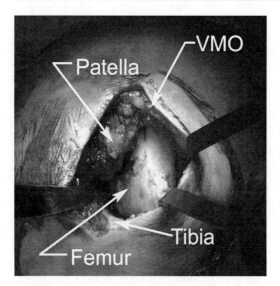

Fig. 3.8 The exposure in flexion. *VMO* vastus medialis oblique

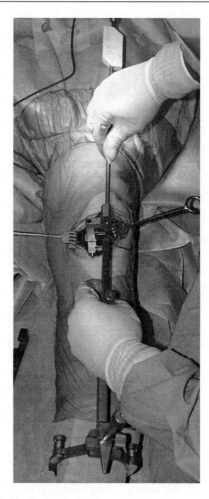

Fig. 3.10 Assemble the tensor device, connecting tower, and rods

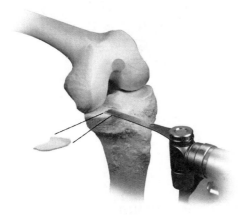

Fig. 3.9 Excise the anterior tibial boss

so as to allow multidirectional adjustments. Now, insert the tibia's square alignment rod into the square hole in the tower by manipulating the tensor and tower with the round femoral rod held proximally (Fig. 3.10).

With that done, align the tibial rod parallel to the tibia in both the AP and lateral planes and tighten the locking screws (Fig. 3.11). So doing determines the orientation but not yet the depth of the tibial cut. The femoral rod should now, in the uncorrected varus knee, project lateral to the marked femoral head. Manually correct the varus

with a valgus stress until the soft tissue tension feels snug. Do not force the knee beyond this point. The femoral rod typically still projects lateral to the femoral head, but only slightly (Fig. 3.12).

While maintaining this manual correction in extension, have an assistant turn the tensor screw to expand the spacer until contact is felt, implying that the space within the joint created with the manipulation is now filled with the spacing device. Release the manual stress to see that the correction is maintained and that the soft tissue tension is not excessive. If satisfied, position a collared screw in the proximal femoral hole and then two uncollared screws (posts) into the tibia.

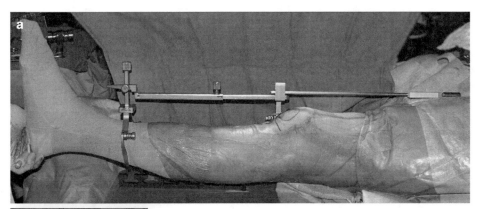

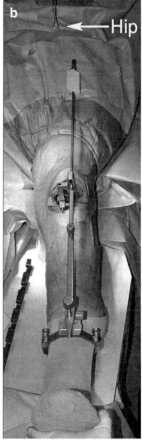

Fig. 3.11 The tibial rod is aligned parallel to the tibia in the (**a**) AP and (**b**) ML planes

Distal Femoral Cut

Remove the tower and rods, leaving the spacer and distal femoral cutting guide in place. Using an angled retractor medially and a skin retractor along the patella, resect the distal femur with the oscillating saw. The knee is in extension so be wary of soft tissue injury as the posterior extent of the cut

is approached. Remove the femoral collared screw, retract the tensor, and slide the tensor off the retained tibial screws (posts) (Fig. 3.13).

Tibial Cuts

While still in extension so as to accommodate a small incision, position the tibial cutting block of

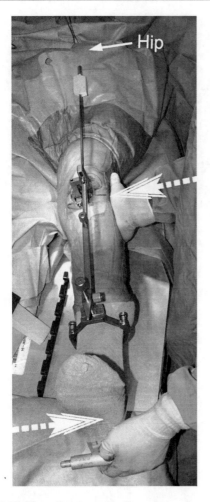

Fig. 3.12 Manually correct the alignment

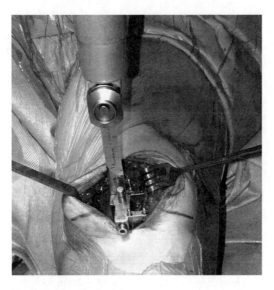

Fig. 3.13 Cut the distal femur

choice (3°, 5°, or 7° slope) at the desired level (8, 10, 12, or 14 mm) and secure it with a Kocher clamp to each uncollared screw (post). Now flex the knee to 90° so as to relax and protect the posterior soft tissues. Manipulate the leg into valgus and external rotation and then position the retractors.

First, with the reciprocating saw blade just inside the notch in the sagittal plane, cut down to the cutting block. Leave the blade in place to serve as a visual and physical guide for the lateral extent of the ensuing cut. Now, with the oscillating saw, make the sloped cut of the tibial plateau between the protected cruciates and MCL (Fig. 3.14a, b).

Flexion and Extension Gaps

The femoral component's sizing and placement keys off the posterior condyle. Therefore, it is important to confirm that the yet-to-be-created flexion gap corresponds to the established extension gap before sizing the femoral component. This is done with the paired extension/flexion gap gauges. If at this time the space is found to be tight, before committing to the posterior condylar cut and its concomitant prosthetic width, open up the flexion gap by shaving off the necessary cartilage and bone from the posterior condyle. Now size the femur. It is easy to adjust the flexion gap before sizing and finishing the femoral cuts. It is difficult to do so afterward (Fig. 3.15a, b).

First check the extension gap with an extension gap gauge. It is the thicker end that is equal to the composite width of a given femoral and tibial implant. Determine the one that is optimal in establishing the desired alignment and soft tissue balance. Presumably and usually this corresponds to the cut chosen for the tibia, that is, 8 or 10 mm as a rule. Whatever composite width is chosen, 8, 10, 12, or 14, be sure the flexion gap then accommodates those projected components by inserting the thinner end of the gauge, the width of which corresponds to the intended tibial component only. If the flexion gap is tight, unless the posterior reference point for the femoral guide is moved anteriorly, the implant when implanted recreates the tight space. Thus, if tight, resect the cartilage and occasionally bone necessary to adequately open up the flexion space.

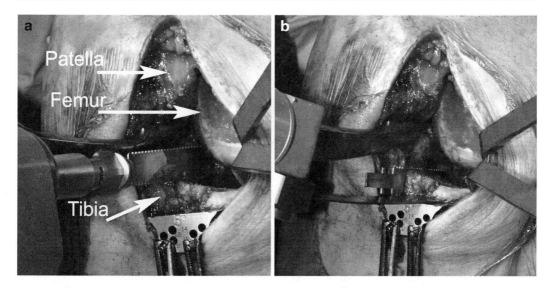

Fig. 3.14 (**a**) With the reciprocating saw just lateral to the medial condyle, cut down to the tibial cutting block. (**b**) Leave the blade in place and protect the MCL with retractors for the oscillating saw cut

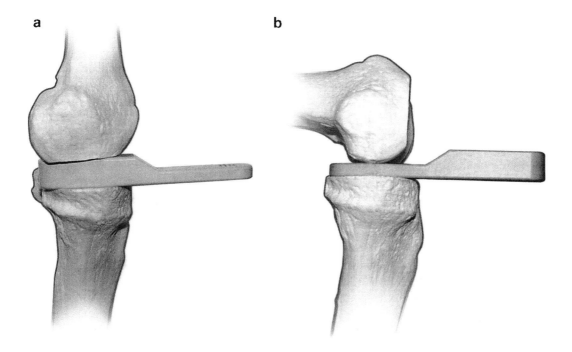

Fig. 3.15 (**a**) Extension and (**b**) flexion gauges

Anterior Femoral Marking

It is time now for sizing and positioning the femoral component. For that to be done accurately requires clear visualization of the entire cut distal surface of the femur. Doing so in flexion is compromised anteriorly by the tight quad and patella. However, while in extension and the quad relaxed, the entire cut surface is readily seen. Taking advantage of this clear view in extension, a mark can be made anteriorly on that cut distal

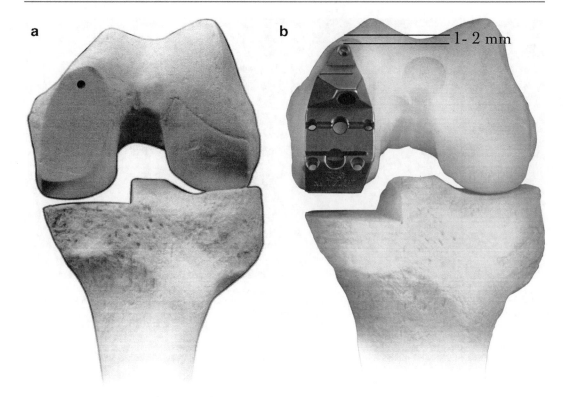

Fig. 3.16 (**a**) Mark the anterior femur at the (**b**) intended screw fixation site

surface that corresponds to where the femoral finishing guide should go. Then, when the knee is next brought into flexion, only this mark need be seen, not the entire distal femoral cut surface. This reduces the need for a more extended division of the quad mechanism or the displacement of the patella (Fig. 3.16a, b).

Also, an advantage of marking the femur in extension for subsequent positioning of the finishing guide is the ability to center the anterior femoral component relative to the cut tibial surface. If the cuts and post holes for the femoral component are centered in extension and then next in flexion relative to the tibial cut surface, the components will be presumably centered upon one another throughout the arc of motion to, thus, avoid edge loading of the tibial plastic.

Femoral Finishing Guide Sizing and Positioning

Having marked the anterior femur with a Bovie or pen in extension, flex the knee to 90° and position the retractors. Choose the femoral finishing guide that, when keyed off the posterior condyle, has an anterior screw hole that corresponds to the mark. If in doubt as to which size fits best, choose the smaller size to avoid having the femoral implant extend beyond the cut femoral surface anteriorly where it might impinge on the patella.

Secure the guide anteriorly with a collared screw through the hole overlying the mark. With the knee still flexed, rotate the posterior aspect of the guide to a position that again centers it over the cut tibial surface. This typically is accomplished by lining up the notch side of the guide to the very edge of the notch side of the femoral cut surface, that is, rotate the guide to the extreme lateral edge of the femoral cut surface. With the guide secured posteriorly with one or two screws, the post holes are drilled, the chamfer cut is made, and then lastly, the posterior condyle. Remove the anterior screw and then the guide with its attached posterior condylar fragment (Fig. 3.17a–d).

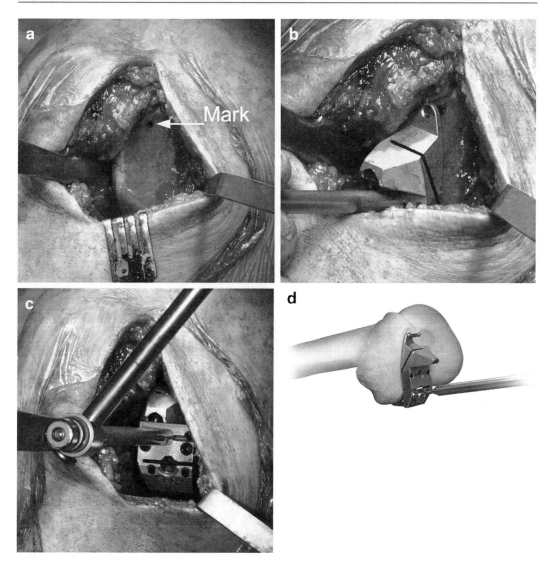

Fig. 3.17 (**a**) The mark is used as (**b**) a target for securing the femoral cutting guide anteriorly before (**c**) pivoting it into position posteriorly and (**d**) securing it with screws

With all cuts now made, visualization of the posterior aspect of the compartment is maximized. First, remove the remaining medial meniscus and then debride the posterior condyle with a curved osteotome to assure an unrestricting flexion recess.

Tibial Sizing and Finishing

Determine optimal coverage of the tibial cut surface with the sizing paddles. If in between sizes, cut away from the tibial spine the small amount necessary to accommodate the larger size. Impact

that provisional plate into place and drill the holes. Impacting the plate will tend to push it posteriorly. Stabilizing the plate first with a short screw anteriorly can prevent this displacement (Fig. 3.18a, b).

Trialing and Cementing

The knee is flexed with the tibial plate in place. With a small incision and a patella that is not displaced, positioning of the trial femoral component, and later the prosthesis, is challenging. It is made easier by flexing the knee to 120° while

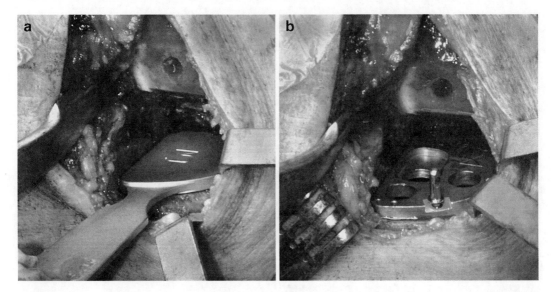

Fig. 3.18 (**a**) Size and (**b**) secure the provisional tibial plate

maintaining a valgus and external rotational stress. With the femoral trial rotated away from the patella, place the longer posterior post into its hole in the femur and impact it slightly. Then slowly extend the knee until the patella is lax enough to allow the trial to be rotated into place beneath it. With the shorter anterior post aligned with its hole, impact the trial fully.

Flexing and stressing the knee once again, slip the plastic trial into place. In extension, the limb alignment should be noted. Of particular importance is to again check that the tissue balance is proper. For a given set of implants, it is thought that in both flexion and extension a valgus stress should produce approximately 2 mm of opening. A 2-mm-wide tension gauge is available. Do not accept a tight space. If all cuts were made in the sequence described, that should not at this point be a problem. Nonetheless, check the tension carefully. Also, check to see that the femoral component tracks centrally over the tibial implant through its arc of motion and confirm that there is no trochlear impingement (Fig. 3.19a–d).

Having checked for debris, cleanse the cut bone surfaces with pulsatile lavage, dry, and then impact over cement the tibial implant with the knee in flexion. A valgus and external rotation stress to the leg improves viewing the

extraction of excess cement using a small curved spatula.

For the femoral component, again flex the knee to 120° and position the femoral implant as previously described. With the posterior post positioned first, extend the knee until the shorter post can be rotated into place and then impacted fully. Remove all excess cement. Now insert the chosen plastic and prop the foot so as to maintain the knee in extension while the cement hardens. Insertion of a drain and closure of the wound can commence at this time (Fig. 3.20).

Conclusion

Implants such as the M/G unicompartmental prosthesis are known to work well for an intermediate time, at least. With improved materials and optimal designs, it is assumed that longer-term success can be achieved. Meanwhile, the challenge is to develop surgical techniques that will further diminish the morbidity of the implantation while enhancing the surgeon's ability to better align and balance the knee. The EM tensor technique using linked femoral and tibial cuts oriented after the alignment and soft tissue correction has been achieved with modestly sized EM instruments is consistent with those goals.

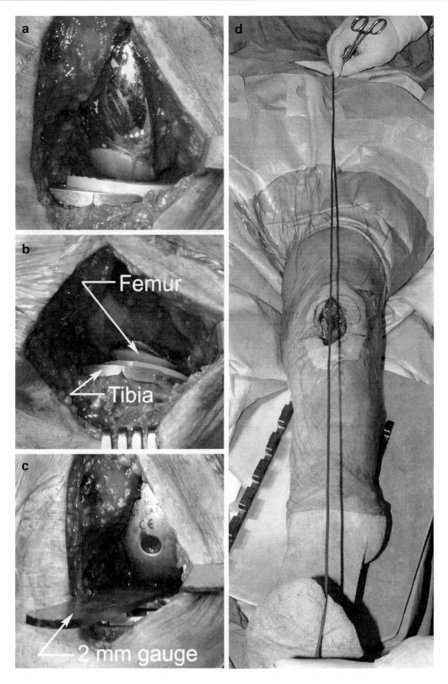

Fig. 3.19 (**a**) The femoral component should be centered over the tibia in both flexion and (**b**) extension. (**c**) Check the tissue tension and (**d**) the limb alignment

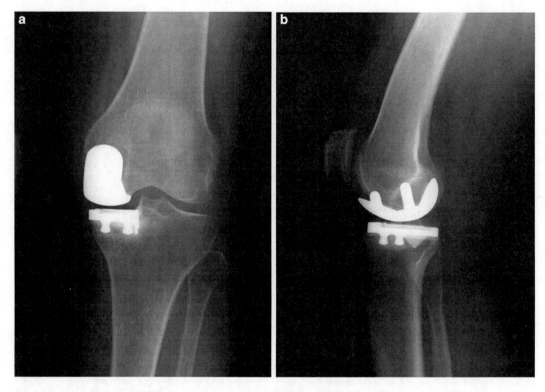

Fig. 3.20 Postoperative (**a**) AP and (**b**) lateral X-ray of an M/G unicompartmental knee

References

1. Caillouette JT. Fat embolism syndrome following the intramedullary alignment guide in total knee arthroplasty. Clin Orthop Relat Res 1990; 251: 198–199
2. Kolettis GT. Safety of one-stage bilateral total knee arthroplasty. Clin Orthop Relat Res 1994; 309:102–109
3. Hasegawa Y, Opishi Y, Shimizu T. Unicompartmental knee arthroplasty for medial gonarthrosis: 5 to 9 years follow-up evaluation of 77 knees. Arch Orthop Trauma Surg [Germany] 1998; 117(4–5): 183–187
4. Murray DW, Goodfellow JW, O'Connor JJ. The Oxford medial unicompartmental arthroplasty: a ten-year survival study. J Bone Joint Surg (Br) 1998; 80(6):983–989
5. Newman JW, Ackroyd DE, Shah NA. Unicompartmental or total knee replacement? Five-year results of a prospective, randomized trial of 102 osteoarthritic knees with unicompartmental arthritis. J Bone Joint Surg (Br) 1998; 80(5):862–865
6. Tabor OB Jr, Tabor OB. Unicompartmental arthroplasty; a long-term follow-up study. J Arthroplasty 1998; 13(4):373–379
7. Marmor L. Unicompartmental knee arthroplasty: ten to thirteen year follow-up study. Clin Orthop Relat Res 1988;226:14
8. Scott RD. Unicompartmental knee arthroplasty. Clin Orthop Relat Res 1991;271:96–100
9. Berger RA, Nedeff DD, Barden RM, et al. Unicompartmental knee arthroplasty: clinical experience at 6- to 10-year follow up. Clin Orthop Relat Res 1999;367:50–60
10. Argenson JN, Chevrol-Benkeddache Y, Aubniac JM. Modern cemented metal-backed unicompartmental knee arthroplasty: a 3 to 10 year follow-up study. 68th annual Meeting of the American Academy of Orthopaedic Surgeons, 2001
11. Pennington DW, Swienckowski JJ, Lutes WB. Unicompartmental knee arthroplasty in patients sixty years of age or younger. J Bone Joint Surg 2003; 85A:1968–1973
12. Laskin RS. Unicompartmental tibiofemoral resurfacing arthroplasty. J Bone Joint Surg 1978;60: 182–185
13. Cartier P, Sanouiller JL, Dreisamer RP. Unicompartmental knee arthroplasty: 10-year minimum follow-up period. J Arthroplasty 1996;11970:782–788
14. Romanowski MR, Repicci JA. Technical aspects of medial versus lateral minimally invasive unicondylar arthroplasty. Orthopedics 2003;26:289–293

Suggested Readings

Philip Gavin. The History Place. http://www.historyplace. com. 4 July 1996

Scott Kurnin. 20th Century Timeline. About. http://www. history1900s.com. February 1997

Joanne Freeman. Timeline of the Civil War. http://www. memory.loc.gov/ammam/cwphtml/cwphone.html. 15 January 2000

MIS Unicondylar Knee Arthroplasty with the Extramedullary Technique*

4

Giles R. Scuderi

Minimally invasive surgery (MIS) unicondylar knee arthroplasty has gained popularity over the recent years following the introduction of the limited approach by Repicci and Eberle [1]. Their limited approach was essentially a freehand technique that used limited instrumentation. Over the years there have been modifications in the surgical instruments in order to perform the procedure accurately and reproducibly through a MIS approach. The Miller Galante Unicondylar prosthesis (Zimmer, Warsaw, IN) introduced intramedullary instrumentation and most recently extramedullary instrumentation [2]. The smaller and reliable modified instruments clearly help in bone preparation and component position producing clinical results that are comparable with a conventional procedure [3, 4]. Improved instrumentation allows the surgeon to operate through a minimally invasive arthrotomy, without everting the patella, and permits more accurate bone

resection. It is the refinements in instrumentation that have contributed to successful clinical results.

General Principles

Alignment in unicondylar knee arthroplasty is determined by femoral and tibial bone resection, and not soft tissue release. Since soft tissue releases to correct deformity are not performed, if the varus or valgus deformity exceeds 15° or if there is a flexion contracture greater than 10°, a total knee arthroplasty should be considered. In unicondylar knee arthroplasty, overcorrection of the knee should be avoided, because this overloads the contralateral compartment and increases the potential for progression of the degenerative arthritis. Reports have shown that slight undercorrection of the knee alignment is correlated with long-term survivorship [5, 6].

The advantage of extramedullary instrumentation in MIS is that it eliminates the need for violation of the femoral intramedullary canal. Extramedullary instruments are designed to provide a means of achieving precision in limb alignment. With the limb aligned in extension, the deformity may be passively corrected. By coupling an extramedullary femoral and tibial guide, the angle of resection for the distal femur and the proximal tibia can be determined, creating a parallel resection of the femur and tibia in extension. The linked cuts are perpendicular to the mechanical axis of the femur and tibia, respectively.

*Adapted from Scuderi GR, Minimally invasive surgery for unicondylar knee arthroplasty: the extramedullary technique, in Scuderi GR, Tria AJ, Berger RA (eds.), *MIS Techniques in Orthopedics*, 2006, with kind permission of Springer Science + Business Media.

G.R. Scuderi (✉)
Insall Scott Kelly Institute for Orthopaedics and Sports Medicine, New York, NY, USA
e-mail: gscuderi@iskinstitute.com

North Shore-LIJ Health System, Great Neck, NY, USA

Albert Einstein College of Medicine,
New York, NY, USA

Approach

The skin incision is made with the knee in flexion and begins from the superior pole of the patella to 1–2 cm distal to the joint line. This straight incision is placed along the medial border of the patella for a medial unicondylar replacement. A limited medial parapatellar capsular arthrotomy is performed, extending from the lower border of the vastus medialis to a point just distal to the joint line along the proximal tibia. To aid visualization, the fat pad is excised along with the anterior horn of the medial meniscus. Subperiosteal dissection is then carried out along the proximal medial tibia, releasing the meniscal tibial attachment, but not releasing the medial collateral ligament. A curved retractor is then placed along the medial tibial border to protect the collateral ligament. Medial tibial and femoral osteophytes are removed along with any osteophytes along the femoral intercondylar notch. With the spacer block technique, the tibia is prepared first [2].

For a lateral unicondylar replacement, the skin incision is made along the lateral border of the patella. The arthrotomy is a lateral capsular incision that extends from the superior pole of the patella, along the lateral border of the patella and patella tendon, and 1–2 cm distal to the joint line. The lateral fat pad can be excised to aid visualization. The meniscal tibial attachment is released and a curved retractor is placed along the lateral border of the tibia. Similar to a medial unicondylar replacement, the tibia will be prepared first.

Tibial Preparation

The tibia is resected with an extramedullary tibial cutting guide. The shaft of the resection guide is set parallel to the tibial shaft. The proximal cutting head is secured to the tibia and the depth and slope of resection is determined. A depth gauge is used so that 2–4 mm of bone is removed from the lowest point on the tibial plateau. Once the desired depth of resection is determined, a retractor is placed medially to protect the medial collateral ligament. With the knee flexed, the proximal tibia is resected (Fig. 4.1). Caution must be taken not

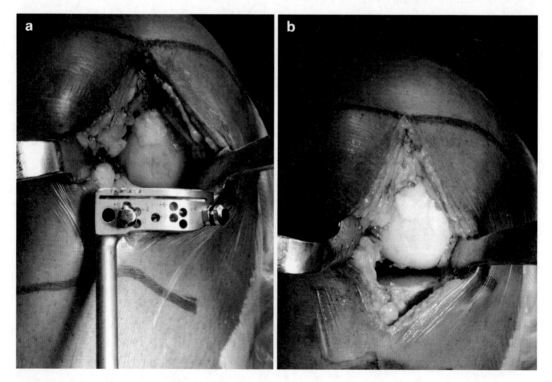

Fig. 4.1 Resection of the proximal tibia with the extramedullary guide (**a**); resected tibia (**b**)

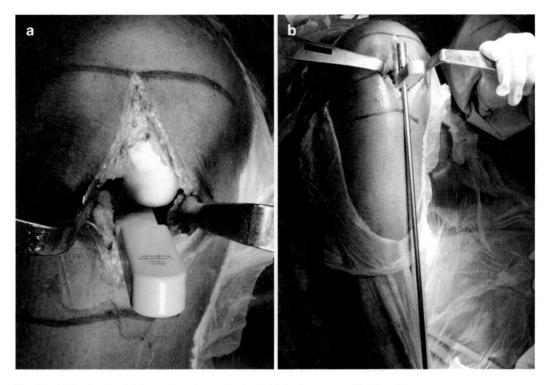

Fig. 4.2 Following the tibial resection, the gap is checked (**a**); alignment rod in place (**b**)

to undercut the attachment of the anterior cruciate ligament and the lateral tibial plateau. With a reciprocating saw, the sagittal tibial cut is made in line with the medial wall of the intercondylar notch down to the level of the transverse cut. The resected tibial bone is then removed. The gap is checked with a spacer block to ensure that appropriate amount of bone has been resected and that the axial alignment is correct (Fig. 4.2). If the gap is too tight with the spacer block in place, additional bone should be resected from the proximal tibia. If the gap is too loose, a thicker spacer block, which correlates to a thicker tibial component, should be inserted.

Femoral Preparation

Following resection of the proximal tibia, the knee is brought into full extension and the 8-mm spacer block, or the appropriately sized spacer block as determined above, is inserted into the joint space. It should be fully inserted and sit flat on the resected tibia to ensure that the proper amount of distal femur will be resected (Fig. 4.3). If there is any difficulty inserting the 8-mm spacer block, then additional bone needs to resected from the proximal tibia. In contrast, if the 8-mm spacer block is too loose, then a thicker spacer block should be inserted.

With the appropriate spacer block in place and the knee in extension, the alignment tower is attached so that the position of the guide can be checked relative to the center of the femoral head (Fig. 4.4). The alignment tower is then removed and the distal femoral resection guide is attached to the spacer block (Fig. 4.5), which is then secured to the distal femur. The distal femur can be resected in full extension, but caution must be taken not to over cut the distal femur and have the saw blade extend beyond the posterior capsule and into the popliteal area. If desired, the femoral cut can be started in extension and finished in flexion. Once the distal femur is resected, the extension gap is checked with a spacer block and alignment rod (Fig. 4.6).

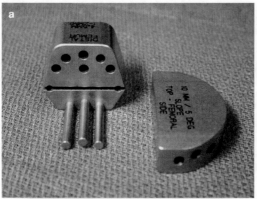

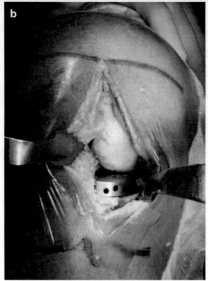

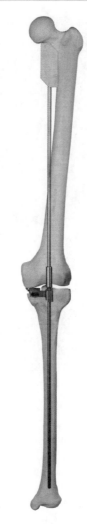

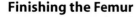
Fig. 4.3 The spacer block (**a**) is inserted into the joint on the resected tibia (**b**)

Fig. 4.4 The alignment tower is attached to the spacer block

Finishing the Femur

Once the extension gap has been determined, the appropriate-sized femoral finishing guide is selected (Fig. 4.7). This guide rests on the flat surface of the distal femur and the posterior extension lies against the posterior condyles. To avoid oversizing the femoral component and causing impingement of the patellofemoral joint, there should be 1–2 mm of exposed bone along the anterior edge of the guide. If the femoral component appears to be in between sizes, it would be preferable to pick the smaller size. The femoral guide should also be rotationally set so that the posterior surface is parallel to the resected tibia. With the guide secured to the femur, the final cuts and lug holes are made. This completes the femoral preparation.

Finishing the Tibia

At this point, the remaining meniscus and osteophytes are removed. The appropriate-sized tibial template, which covers the entire surface without overhang, is selected (Fig. 4.8). The template is secured to the proximal tibia and the lug holes are drilled. The tibial template is left in place for the trial reduction.

Trial Reduction

With the knee in 90° of flexion and a retractor in the intercondylar notch to pull back the patella, the provisional femoral component is seated on

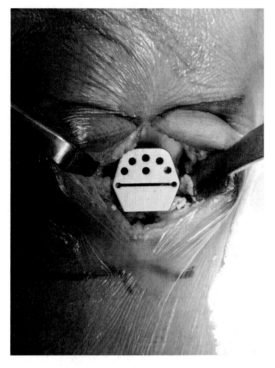

Fig. 4.5 The distal femoral resection guide is attached to the spacer block

the distal femur. A trial tibial articular surface is then placed on the tibial template. With all the provisional components in place, the knee is checked for range of motion and stability. Appropriate soft tissue tension is checked with the 2-mm tension gauge inserted between the femoral component and the tibial articulation (Fig. 4.9). In general, the correct thickness of the tibial prosthesis should allow for approximately 2 mm of joint laxity in full extension.

Final Components

The trial components are removed and the bone surfaces are cleansed with water pick lavage in an effort to remove blood and debris from the surfaces. In preparation for cementing, the bone is dried. The modular tibial component is cemented in place first. With the knee hyperflexed and externally rotated, a small amount of cement is placed on the exposed surface of the tibia. An additional amount of cement is placed on the undersurface of the tibial component. The final tibial component is then pressed into place and the excess cement is removed. To fully seat the tibial component, it is impacted into place and any extruded cement is removed.

With the knee in 90° of flexion, a retractor is placed in the intercondylar notch to hold the

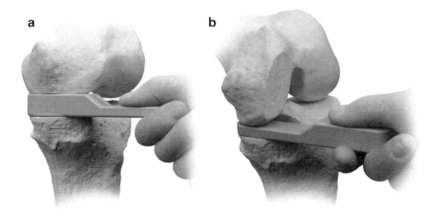

Fig. 4.6 The gaps are checked in extension (**a**), and flexion (**b**)

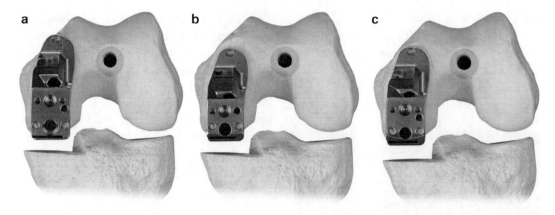

Fig. 4.7 (**a–c**) The correct femoral finishing guide is selected

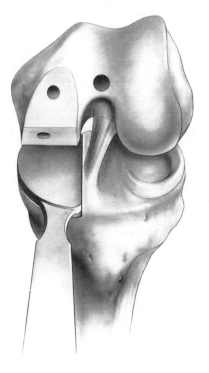

Fig. 4.8 The tibial template is placed on the resected tibia

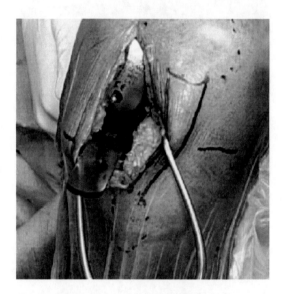

Fig. 4.9 With the provisional components in place, the 2-mm tension gauge is inserted in the joint

patella back so that the femur is exposed. A small amount of cement is placed on the distal femur and along the backside of the femoral component. The femoral component is impacted in place and all excess cement is removed. The modular tibial polyethylene articular surface is then inserted and a final check of motion and stability is performed.

With the final components in place (Fig. 4.10), the knee is irrigated with an antibiotic solution. The arthrotomy, subcutaneous layer and skin are closed in a routine fashion.

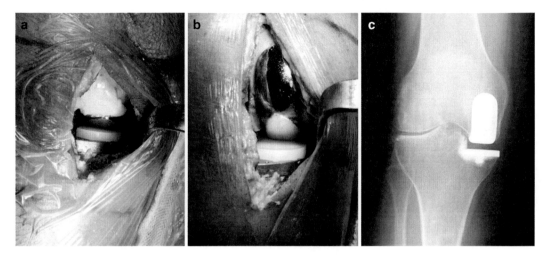

Fig. 4.10 The final components in place (**a**, **b**) with the resultant radiograph (**c**)

Summary

Minimally invasive unicondylar knee arthroplasty implanted with extramedullary instrumentation minimizes soft tissue dissection, does not violate the femoral intramedullary canal, and ensures accurate component positioning. Since the proximal tibial resection and the distal femoral resection are linked in extension, this coupled resection and desired soft tissue tension set limb alignment. The cuts are parallel and result in a preset gap that is calculated to match the thickness of the implants. Gap balancing reduces the need for recutting, will help preserve bone stock, and assures accurate component positioning. Final postoperative alignment is determined by the composite thickness of the components. Reliable instrumentation results in accurate bone resection and component position, which are necessary for a successful clinical outcome.

References

1. Repicci JA, Eberle RW. Minimally invasive surgical technique for unicondylar knee replacement. J South Orthop Assoc 1999;8:20–27
2. Zimmer monograph. The Zimmer unicompartmental high flex knee: intramedullary, spacer block option and extramedullary minimally invasive surgical techniques, 2004
3. Barnes CL, Scott RD. Unicondylar replacement. In: Scuderi GR, Tria AJ, eds Surgical Techniques in Total Knee Arthroplasty. Springer, New York, 2002, 106–111
4. Scuderi GR. Instrumentation for unicondylar knee replacement. In: Scuderi GR, Tria AJ, eds MIS of the Hip and the Knee: A Clinical Perspective. Springer, New York, 2004, 87–104
5. Berger RA, Nedeff DD, Barden RM, et al. Unicompartmental knee arthroplasty: clinical experience at 6- to 10-year follow-up. Clin Orthop 1999; 367:5060
6. Cartier P, Sanouiller JL, Grelsamer RP. Unicompartmental knee arthroplasty: 10-year minimum follow-up period. J Arthroplasty 1996;11:782–788

MIS Arthroplasty with the UniSpacer*

5

Richard H. Hallock

Middle-age osteoarthritis of the knee remains a problem with many treatment options. It can be treated in its earlier stages with a combination of oral medication, intraarticular injection with cortisone or viscosupplementation, physical therapy, and arthroscopic debridement. Once the patient has reached a level of disability that is not responding to these less invasive treatment modalities, the patient and physician are both faced with the decision to choose a more invasive surgical option. The selection of the best surgical alternative will depend on many nonsurgical issues including the patient's age, weight, sex, activity level, and occupation. This decision will also be based on the extent of cartilage degeneration, as well as bony deformity. These options include high tibial osteotomy, unicompartmental knee arthroplasty, total knee arthroplasty, and the UniSpacer. The final decision on which of these techniques is ultimately used will come down to patient and surgeon preference based on the individual set of circumstances.

The UniSpacer was designed on both very traditional orthopedic principles as well as some

nontraditional orthopedic concepts [1–5]. It is a cobalt chrome metallic device that is inserted into the medial compartment of the knee. The bearing surfaces of the device have a metal on cartilage/bone interface on both the femoral and tibial surfaces. Metal on biologic interfaces have been used traditionally in orthopedics in hemiarthroplasty of the shoulder, hemiarthroplasty of the hip, and nonresurfaced patellae in total knee replacement. It serves as a self-centering shim, which replaces the missing articular and meniscal cartilage of the medial compartment.

As such, the thickness of the shim is determined by the amount of missing articular and meniscal cartilage within the constraints of the collateral and cruciate ligaments. The varus deformity will thus only be corrected back to the patient's premorbid knee alignment. This realignment will off load the medial compartment of the knee without over correcting the alignment and accelerating lateral compartment degeneration. What is different about this device from traditional arthroplasty is that it is neither fixed to the bony surfaces of the tibia or the femur, nor requires bone cuts or bone removal for implantation. The geometry of the device with its concave femoral surface and convex tibial surface allows it to function as a self-centering shim between the biological femoral and tibial surfaces of the patient. These nontraditional concepts avoid the traditional modes of arthroplasty failure including loosening, polyethylene wear, and malpositioning of components. As such, it can function either as a final arthroplasty or as a

*Adapted from Hallock RH, MIS Arthroplasty with the UniSpacer, in Scuderi G, Tria A, Berger R (eds), *MIS Techniques in Orthopedics*, New York, Springer, 2006, with kind permission of Springer Science+Business Media, Inc.

R.H. Hallock (✉)
The Orthopedic Institute of Pennsylvania,
Camp Hill, PA, USA
e-mail: rhhallock@aol.com

safe bridge procedure in younger patients, which does not alter the bony and ligamentous anatomy for a next-step procedure.

Preoperative Evaluation

The preoperative evaluation for the UniSpacer requires the same type of evaluation that would be necessary to perform a high tibial osteotomy, unicompartmental knee replacement, or total knee replacement. Routine X-ray evaluation should include anteroposterior (AP) erect views of the knee, which allow evaluation of the loss of joint space as well as the femoral tibial axis (Fig. 5.1). The surgeon should pay particular attention to medial subluxation of the femur relative to the tibia and deformity of the tibial plateau (Fig. 5.2).

Either of these two conditions would preclude the use of the UniSpacer. The lateral X-ray of the knee is necessary to view the relative position of the femoral condyle with respect to the tibia. Anterior translation of the tibia relative to the femur may indicate chronic anterior cruciate ligament

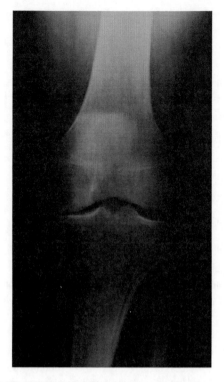

Fig. 5.1 Loss of medial joint space without deformation of the tibia

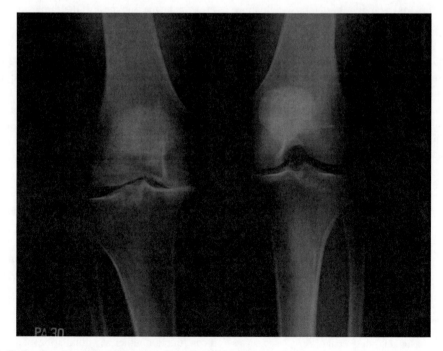

Fig. 5.2 Deformity of the tibia and medial subluxation of the femur

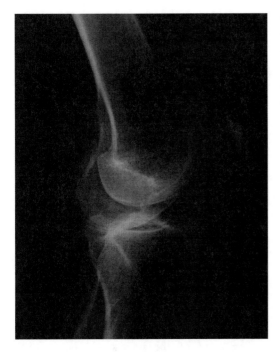

Fig. 5.3 A anterior subluxation of the tibia suggestive of chronic anterior cruciate ligament (ACL) deficiency

insufficiency, which may also be a contraindication for the use of the UniSpacer (Fig. 5.3). The lateral view also demonstrates posterior femoral osteophytes. Large posterior femoral osteophytes can produce a flexion contracture greater than 5°, which is also a contraindication for the use of the UniSpacer. The skyline view is necessary to eval uate the patellofemoral joint. Any significant loss of joint space or osteophyte formation may also contraindicate the use of the UniSpacer, especially if the patient has symptoms, which can be confused medial joint pain. A magnetic resonance imaging (MRI) scan can also be useful in evaluating the status of the knee. Questions concerning the integrity of the anterior cruciate ligament as well as the status of the patella femoral joint can also be answered with an MRI scan.

Surgical Technique

Since the UniSpacer requires no bone cuts and has no fixation, the surgical technique is decidedly different than traditional arthroplasty. The surgical technique focuses on restoring the knee alignment through thorough joint debridement and implantation of an intraarticular shim. This will be broken down into steps including arthrotomy, osteophyte resection and anterior medial meniscectomy, chondroplasty, tweenplasty, sizing, insertion technique, fluoroscopy, and final implantation and closure.

Surgical Preparation

Preoperative antibiotic prophylaxis is utilized on all patients. The use of a thigh tourniquet is optional and left to surgeon preference. The arthroscopy portals and incision line can be infiltrated with local anesthetic with epinephrine to decrease intraoperative bleeding, especially if the patient does not have a tourniquet. The patient is placed in the supine position with the knee prepped and draped in a routine fashion.

Rigid leg holders should be avoided since they will inhibit the surgeon from placing the knee through a range of motion, and they will interfere with use of the fluoroscopy equipment later in the case.

Arthroscopy

Every patient who is considered for the UniSpacer should have an arthroscopy performed either at the time of surgery or during the previous 12 months. Inappropriate candidates can be deselected based on the extent of degeneration present at the time of the arthroscopy. The arthroscopy is also useful with some of the initial debridement necessary to proceed with insertion of the UniSpacer. An initial evaluation of the patellofemoral joint, lateral compartment including the lateral meniscus, as well as the cruciate ligament complex should be performed. Any significant degeneration in the patellofemoral compartment or the lateral compartment should result in deselection of the current UniSpacer candidate. Mild grade I to grade II chondromalacia of the patellofemoral joint and lateral compartment is acceptable. Any grade of chondromalacia worse than that degree of degeneration should lead to deselection of that patient for a UniSpacer. Since an intact lateral compartment, including an intact lateral meniscus, is critical when weight bearing is going to be shifted to that compartment, every patient should have an intact lateral meniscus as well as only mild chondromalacic changes involving the lateral femoral condyle and lateral tibial plateau. It is very difficult to distinguish anteromedial knee pain originating from the medial compartment versus the patellofemoral joint. Any patient with significant degeneration involving the patella or femoral sulcus also should be deselected. The cruciate ligament complex also needs to be thoroughly examined.

Many of these patients have had previous arthrotomies for medial meniscectomy as a result of old injuries. When that occurs, the cruciate ligament complex should be examined for complete integrity of both the anterior and the posterior cruciate ligaments. Any patient with deficiency of either the anterior or posterior cruciate ligament will require either reconstruction of these ligaments or consideration of other treatment options. The most common reason for deselection of any UniSpacer candidate is evaluation of the medial compartment. Most UniSpacer candidates have bipolar degenerative disease involving both the femoral condyle and tibial plateau. If the patient has deformity of the tibial plateau subchondral bone plate resulting in remodeling of the medial edge of the tibial plateau, that patient should also be deselected. When this occurs, the tibial plateau has essentially a convex surface instead of the normal shallow, concave surface for the UniSpacer to translate on (Fig. 5.4). Any convex surface of the tibial plateau will inhibit normal translational and rotatory motion that is required for restoration of normal knee kinematics. If, after initial arthroscopic evaluation, the patient is considered to be a satisfactory candidate for utilization of the UniSpacer, several of the initial debridement steps can be performed arthroscopically. This includes resection of the posterior horn of the medial meniscus. The medial meniscus is usually degenerated in these patients, and completion of the posterior meniscectomy can be performed arthroscopically back to the junction of

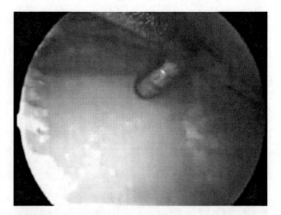

Fig. 5.4 Medial tibial bone loss, which cannot be contoured to create normal UniSpacer kinematics. The subchondral bone has been remodeled to create a convex surface

the red and white zones. Any residual leading edge of the meniscus should be resected as this can result in translation of the UniSpacer over the leading edge of the meniscus. The residual boundary of the meniscus will act as a partial physical constraint. Once the posterior meniscectomy has been completed, the evaluation of the intercondylar osteophytes can proceed. It is not unusual for osteophytes to form in the intercondylar regions in these patients.

Osteophytes abrading the anterior cruciate ligament can cause degeneration of an intact anterior cruciate ligament and eventually result in incompetency. These osteophytes adjacent to the anterior cruciate ligament should be resected if visualized arthroscopically. The osteophytes on the lateral/posterior aspect of the medial femoral condyle can also be difficult to visualize after the arthroscopy has been performed. If that is the case, it is often easier to resect these osteophytes using the aid of the arthroscope. Again, the goal of osteophyte resection adjacent to the intercondylar notch is to restore normal cruciate ligament excursion in addition to removing any abnormal femoral anatomy that may cause aberrant UniSpacer motion.

Arthrotomy

The arthrotomy for insertion of the UniSpacer is very similar to the arthrotomy performed for

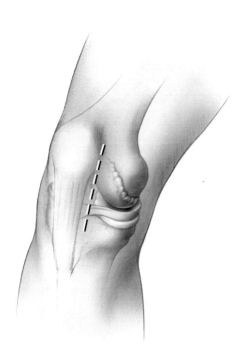

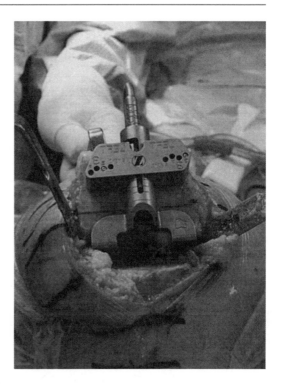

Fig. 5.5 A medial parapatellar incision from mid-patella to the tibial joint line (From Hallock RH, MIS arthroplasty with the UniSpacer. In: Scuderi G, Tria A, Berger R (eds.), *MIS Techniques in Orthopedics*, New York, Springer, 2006, with kind permission of Springer Science and Business Media, Inc.)

Fig. 5.6 A mobile window to the medial compartment with release of the anteromedial corner of the proximal tibia (From Hallock RH, MIS arthroplasty with the UniSpacer. In: Scuderi G, Tria A, Berger R (eds.), *MIS Techniques in Orthopedics*, New York, Springer, 2006, with kind permission of Springer Science and Business Media, Inc.)

insertion of a traditional unicompartmental arthroplasty. The incision usually extends from the mid patella down to the tibial joint line (Fig. 5.5). The subcutaneous tissue is undermined to allow a mobile view of the medial compartment. The medial retinaculum is incised from the superior pole of the patella down to the proximal tibia. The anteromedial corner of the knee is released, including transection of the anterolateral horn of the medial meniscus. Subperiosteal release of the proximal 2 cm of the tibia should be performed when it is necessary to resect osteophytes off of the medial aspect of the tibia (Fig. 5.6). This release is not necessary when there is only minimal medial tibial osteophyte formation present. The arthrotomy should allow visualization of the medial facet of the patella, intercondylar notch, medial femoral condyle, and medial tibial plateau when necessary. A small portion of the infrapatellar fat pad can be resected

when visualization of the intercondylar notch or medial compartment is impaired with just the medial arthrotomy.

Osteophyte Resection and Anteromedial Meniscectomy

Following the arthrotomy, a complete debridement of medial compartment osteophytes is necessary to allow full excursion of the medial collateral and cruciate ligament complex. Initially, any overhanging osteophytes adjacent to the medial aspect of the patella should be resected. Osteophytes are frequently present along the medial border of the patella. When the femoral tibial axis is corrected from varus to valgus alignment, these osteophytes can impinge on the medial aspect of the femoral sulcus. It is imperative to debride these osteophytes

a   b

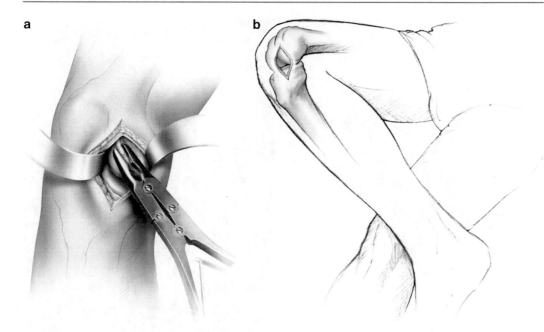

Fig. 5.7 The Fig.-of-four position necessary to resect osteophytes from the posterior region of the medial femoral condyle (From Hallock RH, MIS arthroplasty with the UniSpacer. In: Scuderi G, Tria A, Berger R (eds.), *MIS Techniques in Orthopedics*, New York, Springer, 2006, with kind permission of Springer Science and Business Media, Inc.)

to avoid residual medial patellofemoral pain. Osteophytes are then resected completely from the anterior aspect of the femoral condyle to the posterior aspect of the femoral condyle. This can be performed usually using a rongeur. The osteophytes need to be resected down to the original borders of the femur.

A retractor is supplied with the instrumentation to allow resection of the posterior osteophyte formation on the femoral condyle (Fig. 5.7). This is most easily accomplished by placing the knee in the figure of four position with the knee flexed. An osteotome can be utilized to shear off the posterior osteophytes to restore the original bony contours. It is also imperative to resect any significant osteophyte formation along the medial border of the tibial plateau. When this occurs, it is necessary to release the deep fibers of the medial collateral ligament and meniscal tibial ligament along the proximal 2-cm region of the tibial plateau. Once this is released, osteophytes can easily be resected that overhang the medial border of the original tibial plateau. It is not unusual for the anterior and middle thirds of the medial meniscus to remain relatively intact in these patients. When this occurs, an open anteromedial meniscectomy should be performed at the level of the junction of the red and white zones to avoid any impingement of the UniSpacer on a residual leading edge of the meniscus. Leaving the red zone of the meniscus intact will create a stable border for the UniSpacer. The surgeon should be careful not to violate the superficial fibers of the medial collateral ligament during this procedure.

Chondroplasty

The degenerative surfaces of the femoral condyle and tibial plateau typically have irregular shapes created by variations in the thickness of the remaining articular cartilage. The tibial surface of the UniSpacer has a uniform, shallow convexity despite the size of the device. In an effort to create the most conformal surface that articulates against the UniSpacer, it is necessary to contour the patient's femoral condyle and tibial plateau.

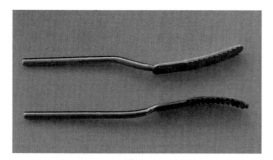

Fig. 5.8 The rasps are shown, which are available to contour the femoral and tibial surfaces to restore a smooth articular surface

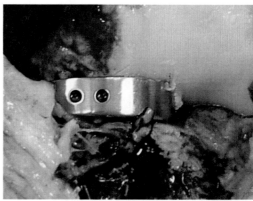

Fig. 5.9 A UniSpacer in position without a proper tweenplasty. Note the impingement on the femoral condyle (From Hallock RH, MIS arthroplasty with the UniSpacer. In: Scuderi G, Tria A, Berger R (eds.), *MIS Techniques in Orthopedics*, New York, Springer, 2006, with kind permission of Springer Science and Business Media, Inc.)

This femoral and tibial "sculpting" will ultimately create the best fit and sizing for the UniSpacer. The surgeon must, therefore, attempt to recreate the anatomic J-curve of the femoral condyle in addition to recreating the shallow dish curvature of the tibial plateau. Despite the fact that the UniSpacer will span cartilage defects on either of these surfaces, it is best to restore the most uniform surfaces, which, ultimately, distributes the load over a greater surface area during loading. Convex and concave rasps are provided with the instrumentation that can be utilized to restore a "best fit" contour to the patient's biological surfaces. The rasps are utilized to smooth out divoted regions of the patient's articular surfaces in addition to restoring more uniform thickness to the remaining articular cartilage (Fig. 5.8). This process is necessary to create more stable kinematics for the UniSpacer during its normal translational/rotational motion. This often requires smoothing out ridges of articular cartilage that create an impediment to normal motion. Areas of full thickness articular cartilage may tend to exaggerate normal motion of the UniSpacer. This is most often seen on the posterior aspect of the femoral condyle where full thickness cartilage often remains. The concave rasp can be used to thin this remaining articular cartilage to avoid an exaggerated posterior translation of the device during flexion.

Although it is not necessary for the surgeon to create a fully conformal surface to the UniSpacer in extension, any attempt to do so will decrease the patient's recovery time. Increased conformity

ultimately leads to distribution of medial compartment load over a greater surface area. This is confirmed when evaluating the clinical results that show improvement occurs not only during the first postoperative year, but also show improvement continues to occur during the second postoperative year.

Tweenplasty

There is one special area that needs to be addressed during the contouring procedure to allow normal anterior rotation of the UniSpacer in full extension. This area, the junction of Whitesides line and the superior aspect of the intercondylar notch, is critical in allowing normal anterior rotation of the UniSpacer in full extension. Since the UniSpacer is driven by the femoral condyle toward the femoral sulcus in full extension, this area needs to be recessed to allow normal rotational motion.

Full-thickness cartilage just above the intercondylar notch must be removed to allow the anterior flange of the device to "screw home" in full extension. If this cartilage is not removed, the UniSpacer will be driven out into an anteromedial position causing impingement and pain during full extension (Fig. 5.9). The degree of articular degeneration on the femoral surface of the patient will dictate how deep this recess needs to be. Most patients require removal of full-thickness articular cartilage in this zone.

Sizing

The UniSpacer comes in six different sizes with respect to length/width and four different thicknesses for each knee. Thus, both the left and right knee each have 24 different-sized implants. The AP length of the device remains proportional to the medial/lateral width of the device as the size increases and decreases. Thus the dimensions of the device increase and decrease proportionally relative to the size. Standard sets range in size between 38 mm in length and 58 mm in length. The device also comes in four varying thicknesses from 2 to 5 mm. Initially, the size of the device is estimated by measuring the AP length of the tibia.

The ultimate sizing, however, is determined by the remaining contour of the femoral condyle. The femoral surface of the UniSpacer must have a radius that is greater than or equal to the surface remaining on the contoured femoral condyle. In other words, the femoral condyle must fit the femoral surface of the UniSpacer without producing any edge loading anteriorly or posteriorly as this creates impingement and eventually may lead to pain or dislocation.

Sizing the Implant

The size of the implant that is ultimately chosen is based on length and thickness. The implant must restore the joint space of the medial compartment that corrects the axial alignment. There is a thickness gauge with the instrument set that can be used to help determine the appropriate thickness. The thickness gauge comes in four different thicknesses ranging from 2 to 5 mm, in 1-mm increments. This gauge is placed between the medial femoral condyle and tibial plateau in both flexion and extension. The correct thickness implant will retension the medial collateral ligament and anterior cruciate ligament while allowing

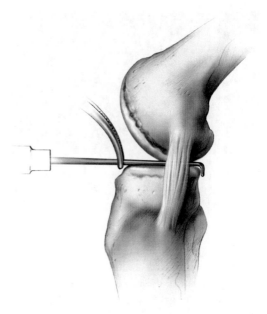

Fig. 5.10 The length initial measurement for the UniSpacer taken off the AP dimension of the tibial plateau (From Hallock RH, MIS arthroplasty with the UniSpacer. In: Scuderi G, Tria A, Berger R (eds.), *MIS Techniques in Orthopedics*, New York, Springer, 2006, with kind permission of Springer Science and Business Media, Inc.)

full extension and maximum flexion. The thickness gauge gives the surgeon an initial trial size that may have to be modified after initial implant testing. The implant must ultimately be sized to fit the contour of the femoral condyle, however, the initial length measurement is taking from the AP dimension of the tibia. An arthroscopy probe is used to hook the posterior aspect of the tibial plateau and then mark the anterior aspect of the tibia using a hemostat (Fig. 5.10). There is a ruler with the instruments that can then be used to check the AP dimension off of the arthroscopy hook. This gives the surgeon an initial trial size with respect to length.

Once the initial measurements have been taken with respect to length and thickness, an implant trial is selected out of the set. The trial is placed on the insertion handle, and then implanted into the medial compartment. The final sizing is actually confirmed by evaluation of the conformity of the femoral surface of the UniSpacer to the femoral condyle. Once the implant is in place, the knee

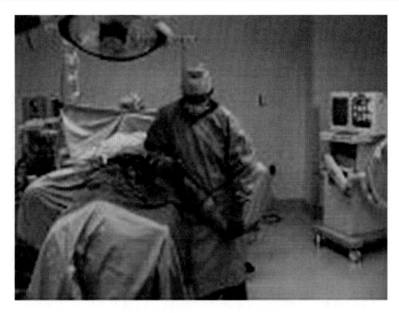

Fig. 5.11 Proper surgeon positioning for UniSpacer insertion (From Hallock RH, MIS arthroplasty with the UniSpacer. In: Scuderi G, Tria A, Berger R (eds.), *MIS* *Techniques in Orthopedics*, New York, Springer, 2006, with kind permission of Springer Science and Business Media, Inc.)

should be placed through a vigorous range of motion to ensure that the UniSpacer has both uniform translation and rotation during flexion and extension cycles. In extension, the UniSpacer should always translate and rotate toward the intercondylar notch, and demonstrate a small amount of anterior overhand off of the tibia. In flexion, the UniSpacer should rotate around the tibial spine, and translate posteriorly, and will frequently show posterior translation off of the tibia.

Insertion Technique

The insertion of both the UniSpacer trials as well as the final implant is often the most intimidating portion of the procedure to learn. Once this technique is mastered, however, it is relatively simple and reproducible. The handle of the testing device allows 360° of rotation, which allows the surgeon to choose the most optimal position of the handle to avoid impingement on the soft tissues during insertion. During the insertion, the trial is tucked into the

medial compartment underneath the medial edge of the patella. With the knee flexed to approximately 45–60°, a valgus stress is applied to the knee and the UniSpacer is held against the femoral condyle with the testing handle. Using some posterior pressure on the handle in addition to a small wiggle, the knee is pulled into full extension and the UniSpacer will drop into the medial compartment. The surgeon must be careful to exert pressure that is directly posterior on the tibial plateau to allow the device to slide into position (Fig. 5.11). The most common error during this technique is improper insertion angle, which results in driving the UniSpacer into the tibial spine instead of into a posterior position on the tibial plateau. Once in position, the implant should center itself under the femoral condyle. To remove the trial implant from the knee, the reverse of this technique is performed. The knee is held in extension with a valgus stress applied to the knee. With the UniSpacer held against the femoral condyle, the knee is flexed. With that maneuver, the UniSpacer can easily be removed from the medial compartment.

Fluoroscopy

It is necessary to confirm correct implant sizing and motion using fluoroscopic guidance. Fluoroscopy allows the surgeon to check the size of the implant relative to the femoral condyle, again ensuring that the UniSpacer has the most anatomic fit to the femoral condyle without undersizing the implant. Fluoroscopy also allows the surgeon to view the motion of the device through normal range of motion. In the fully extended position, the UniSpacer should translate several millimeters anterior to the tibial plateau on the lateral view (Fig. 5.12). In flexion, the UniSpacer should translate to the posterior aspect of the tibia or extend several millimeters past the posterior aspect of the tibial plateau (Fig. 5.13). On the AP view in full extension, the UniSpacer should appear rotated with the anterior horn of the UniSpacer rotated centrally toward the tibial spine. As the surgeon becomes more comfortable with the technique, the fluoroscopy can be kept to a minimum.

Final Implantation and Closure

Once the optimum implant size has been selected, and fluoroscopy is completed, the final implant is inserted into the medial compartment. The handle of the insertion tool is slightly different than the testing tool. The implant is connected to the insertion handle using converging pins. These pins are more fragile than the large pin on the anterior aspect of the trial implants. The insertion technique, however, is basically the same. Once the final implant is in position, the surgeon should place the knee through a range of motion to confirm proper kinematics. The wound is closed in a standard fashion using heavier suture material in the deeper retinacular layer and the routine subcutaneous and skin closure preferred by the surgeon. Patients do not require immobilization unless the surgeon feels the patient would have improved initial ambulation with the extra support.

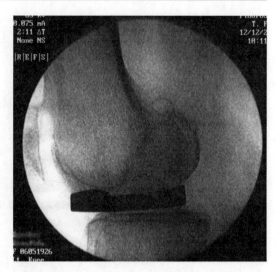

Fig. 5.12 Lateral fluoroscopy view with the knee extended. Note the anterior position of the UniSpacer on the tibial plateau

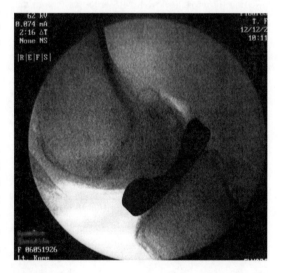

Fig. 5.13 A lateral fluoroscopy view with the knee flexed. Note the posterior translation of the UniSpacer on the tibial plateau. The UniSpacer follows the femoral condyle during femoral roll back

References

1. Hallock RH, Fell BM. Unicompartmental tibial hemiarthroplasty: early results of the UniSpacer knee. Clin Orthop Relat Res. 2003 Nov;(416):154–63
2. Hallock RH. The UniSpacer knee system: have we been there before? Orthopedics. 2003;26(9):9534

3. Geier KA. UniSpacer for knee osteoarthritis. Orthop Nurs. 2003;22(5):369–70

4. Friedman MJ. UniSpacer. Arthroscopy. 2003 Dec; 19(Suppl 1):120–1

5. Dressler K, Ellermann A. [UNISPACER - a new minimally-invasive therapeutic concept for the isolated medial knee joint disease]. Z Orthop Ihre Grenzgeb. 2004;142(2):131–3

MIS Total Knee Arthroplasty with the Limited Medial Parapatellar Arthrotomy

6

Giles R. Scuderi

Minimally invasive (MIS) total knee arthroplasty (TKA) has become a popular procedure with surgeons using a variety of surgical exposures including the limited medial parapatellar arthrotomy, also known as the limited quadriceps-splitting approach; the midvastus approach; the subvastus approach; and the quadriceps-sparing approach [1]. The limited medial parapatellar arthrotomy is a versatile approach that can be easily converted to a traditional approach if necessary. Advantages of this technique include diminished postoperative morbidity, less postoperative pain, decreased blood loss, and an earlier functional recovery [2–5]. However, while limiting the exposure in MIS, the integrity of the TKA must not be compromised. Following specific guidelines in patient selection and surgical technique, the clinical outcome can be predictable.

MIS TKA is not for every patient or for every surgeon. Patient selection is critical and it has been observed that thin female patients with minimal deformity and good preoperative range of motion were ideal candidates for MIS TKA [1, 5]. There is a gender bias with 71% of female subjects compared with 33% of male subjects

being suitable candidates for the MIS TKA. Contributing to this gender difference is that male muscular patients with large femurs tended to be better served with a standard medial parapatellar arthrotomy. Furthermore, a broader femoral transepicondylar width dictates a longer skin incision and arthrotomy [5]. It has also been observed that when considering patients for a MIS TKA, they tend to be of shorter stature and lighter weight. When it comes to the variable of weight, realize that it is the distribution of the weight and the quality of the fat that are also contributing factors. While an obese patient with long thin legs, soft fat and elastic skin may be eligible for MIS TKA; short heavy legs with brawny skin are not ideal candidates. In the final analysis of female patients and weight it has been reported [5] that the average body mass index (BMI) was significantly smaller in the MIS group (<30 kg/mm [2]).

The degree of deformity affects the extent of the surgical exposure. Knees with severe fixed angular deformities often require extensive soft tissue releases and may not be ideal for MIS TKA. Therefore, it is recommended that the MIS procedure be limited to knees with <15° of varus or <20° of valgus. Additionally, since the knee will have to be positioned into various angles of knee flexion during the procedure, it is recommended that the knee have an arc of motion of 90° and a flexion contracture <10° [1, 5]. Preoperative radiographs can be used to determine the patella height and length of the patella tendon. Patella infera, as determined by the Insall

G.R. Scuderi (✉)
Insall Scott Kelly Institute for Orthopaedics and Sports Medicine, New York, NY, USA
e-mail: gscuderi@iskinstitute.com

North Shore-LIJ
Health System, Great Neck, NY, USA

Albert Einstein College of Medicine,
New York, NY, USA

Salvati ratio or Blackburn–Peel ratio, may pose technical difficulties in exposing the joint and laterally subluxing the patella. Therefore, if the patella tendon is short and patella infera is present, it is recommended that the arthrotomy be extended further into the quadriceps tendon, avoiding injury to the patella tendon or avulsion at the tibial tubercle.

The integrity of the skin must not be compromised and, for that reason, patients with rheumatoid or inflammatory arthritis must be approached with caution. Many of these patients have thin, friable skin that can easily tear, so it is better to control the length of the incision by sharp dissection and avoid an intraoperative traumatic injury. Additionally, it is not uncommon for a rheumatoid knee to have abundant hypertrophic inflammatory synovitis, which needs to be removed. In order to perform a complete synovectomy of all compartments, it is recommended that these knees be approached with a standard medial parapatellar arthrotomy. Finally, care must be taken not to place too much tension on the supporting structures in the presence of inflammatory arthritis, especially if associated with generalized osteopenia. Overzealous retraction may result in direct injury to the ligaments, avulsion injuries, or, worse, fracture. Therefore, for these cases, it is recommended that a traditional approach be performed.

Finally, when it comes to patient selection, there are several final variables that need to be considered, including hypertrophic osteoarthritis, prior surgical procedures, and complexity of the arthroplasty. In the presence of exuberant osteophyte formation around the femur, the osteophytes should be removed early during the exposure when performing a MIS approach. This enhances visualization of the joint and positioning of the retractors. Prior surgical procedures pose several problems, including incorporation of prior skin incisions, hardware removal, bone defects, loss of motion, and deformity. In dealing with complex cases that require bone grafting or component augmentation, an extensile approach should be employed. Following the recommendations detailed above, the ideal patient for a MIS TKA can be determined.

Surgical Technique

The limited medial parapatellar arthrotomy is the most versatile of the MIS approaches because it has evolved from a traditional approach performed by most surgeons [6]. The learning curve for this technique is short as surgeons gradually reduce the length of the skin incision and the arthrotomy into the quadriceps tendon in order to gain exposure of the knee joint. With lateral subluxation of the patella, instead of eversion, both the femur and tibia can be visualized without extending the arthrotomy high into the quadriceps tendon. Exposure and placement of the instrumentation does require placing the knee in various position of knee flexion through out the procedure, as well as careful placement of the retractors by the surgical assistant. Some key points are detailed in the following discussion.

The limb is prepped and draped free in the usual sterile fashion. The surgical assistants stabilize the leg with a sand bag placed at the foot of the table. Specialized leg-holding devices may be used but are not mandatory. A straight anterior midline incision is made in extension, extending from the superior aspect of the tibial tubercle to the superior border of the patella. The skin incision is made as small as possible in every patient, but is extended as needed during the procedure to allow for adequate visualization and avoidance of excess skin tension. One intraoperative observation pertaining to the skin incision is the U sign and the V sign. If the skin is under a great deal of tension, the proximal and distal apex will form a U or possibly even flatten out (Fig. 6.1a). This may have a tendency to tear if put under further tension and should be lengthened. Skin under the appropriate tension should form a V at the apices (Fig. 6.1b) [6]. Full-thickness medial and lateral flaps are created over the extensor mechanism. Release of the deep fascia proximally beneath the skin and superficial to the quadriceps tendon facilitates mobilization of the skin and enhances exposure. With the knee in flexion and due to the elasticity of the skin, the incision will stretch an average of 3.75 cm from extension to flexion [5].

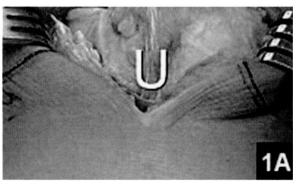
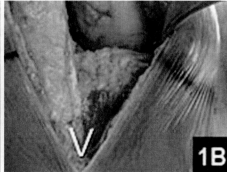

Fig. 6.1 (**a–c**) The skin incision under tension will form the U sign (**a**); minimal skin tension will form the V sign (**b**) (From Scuderi GR, Patient-based MIS TKA: for everything there is a season, OrthoSupersite, http://www.orthosupersite.com/view.asp?rID = 31438. Copyright © 2008 SLACK, Incorporated.)

In an attempt to reduce intraoperative and postoperative bleeding, the quadriceps tendon, along the path of the arthrotomy and the medial retinaculum is injected with 1% lidocaine and epinephrine. This technique has shown a significant reduction in postoperative bleeding. In a comparison study, the average postoperative hemoglobin drop was 3.37 g/dL for the standard approach and 2.05 g/dL for the mini-incision with epinephrine injection [7]. The limited medial parapatellar arthrotomy is a shortened version of the traditional approach (Fig. 6.2). The arthrotomy is of a sufficient length to sublux the patella laterally over the lateral femoral condyle without eversion. In most cases, the incision into the quadriceps tendon extends 2–4 cm above the superior pole of the patella. If there is difficulty displacing the patella laterally or if the patella tendon is at risk of injury, the arthrotomy is extended proximally until adequate exposure can be achieved.

Once the exposure is achieved, the bone preparation begins with the knee flexed at 90°, and retractors are placed both medially and laterally to help aid in exposure, avoid undue skin tension, and to protect the collateral ligaments and the patella tendon. In order to aid visualization and avoid undue tension to the skin, the surgical assistants are instructed in proper placement of retractors and positioning of the knee. This creates a mobile window of exposure (Fig. 6.3). With experience, it will become obvious that the bone

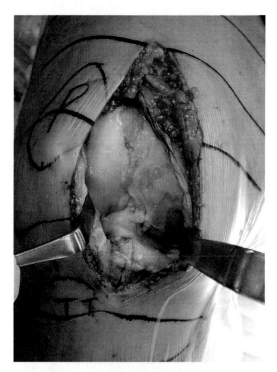

Fig. 6.2 The limited medial parapatellar arthrotomy (From Scuderi GR, Tria AJ, Jr., Minimal incision total knee arthroplasty. In: Scuderi GR, Tria AJ, Jr. (eds.), *MIS of the Hip and the Knee*. New York: Springer, 2004, with kind permission of Springer Science + Business Media, Inc.)

preparation and resection is performed at different angles of knee flexion. In addition, as the bone is resected from the proximal tibia and distal femur, there is more flexibility to the soft tissue envelope and greater exposure is achieved.

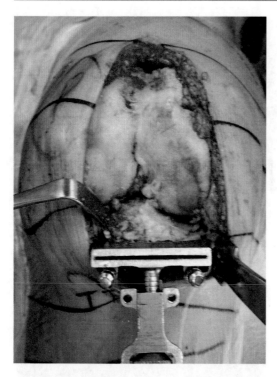

Fig. 6.3 The limited arthrotomy is actually a mobile window (From Scuderi GR, Tria AJ, Jr., Minimal incision total knee arthroplasty. In: Scuderi GR, Tria AJ, Jr. (eds.), *MIS of the Hip and the Knee*. New York: Springer, 2004, with kind permission of Springer Science + Business Media, Inc.)

For the limited medial parapatellar approach and other MIS approaches, smaller instruments have been developed. These smaller instruments, such as the modified 4-in-1 multi-referencing instruments (Zimmer, Warsaw, IN) are advantageous. Although the instrumentation has been modified, there is no difference in the surgical technique. However, since the instruments are reduced in size, care must be taken to make sure they are securely fixed to the bone. Screw fixation, in contrast to smooth nails, is more secure and is used routinely. In addition, the saw blades are narrower to avoid impingement in the modified instruments.

The order of bone resection is dependent upon the surgeon's preference, but I recommend cutting the tibia first because the removal of bone from the proximal tibia will impact both the flexion and extension gap, thereby facilitating preparation of the femur. Tibial resection is accomplished with the assistance of an extramedullary guide that is side specific and medially biased (Fig. 6.4). The tibial guide is centered on the tibial tubercle and set at the appropriate depth and angle of resection. As mentioned earlier, the assistants are carefully protecting the supporting soft tissue structures during the bone resection.

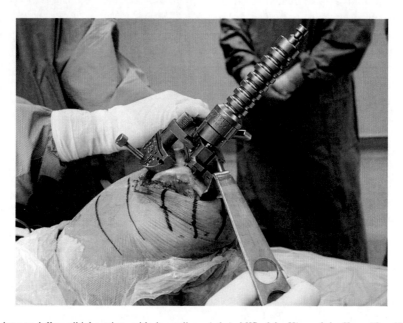

Fig. 6.4 The intramedullary tibial cutting guide is medially offset (From Scuderi GR, Tria AJ, Jr., Minimal incision total knee arthroplasty. In: Scuderi GR, Tria AJ, Jr. (eds.), *MIS of the Hip and the Knee*. New York: Springer, 2004, with kind permission of Springer Science + Business Media, Inc.)

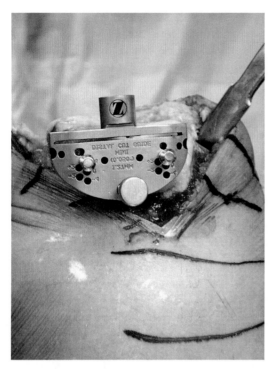

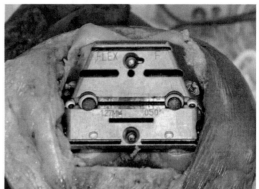

Fig. 6.6 The AP cutting guide

Fig. 6.5 The distal femoral cutting guide (From Scuderi GR, Tria AJ, Jr., Minimal incision total knee arthroplasty. In: Scuderi GR, Tria AJ, Jr. (eds.), *MIS of the Hip and the Knee*. New York: Springer, 2004, with kind permission of Springer Science + Business Media, Inc.)

Following resection of the proximal tibia and removal of the bone, attention is directed to the distal femur. An intramedullary femoral cutting guide is inserted into the distal femur, which is resected with the appropriate degree of valgus, as determined during the preoperative planning (Fig. 6.5). Once this is completed, the femur is sized and the rotational axis of the femur is determined. The femoral rotation can be set along the anteroposterior (AP) axis, the epicondylar axis, or a predetermined rotation based upon surgical preference. Sizing of the femur is based upon the surgeon's preference, the measured AP anatomy, and the type of prosthesis. When the AP dimension is in between sizes and a cruciate-retaining prosthesis is being implanted, the surgeon may downsize the prosthesis. In contrast, with a posterior-stabilized prosthesis, the surgeon may upsize the component or pick the implant size that is closest to the measured anatomy. In either case, the chosen AP cutting block is secured in the appropriate degree of external rotation and the bone is resected (Fig. 6.6).

Once the femur and tibial bone are resected, laminar spreaders are used to distract the knee joint at 90° of flexion. Since it is my preference to implant a posterior-stabilized knee prosthesis, both cruciate ligaments along with the medial and lateral menisci are removed. For surgeons who prefer a posterior cruciate-retaining design, the mini-incision approach provides adequate exposure and the posterior cruciate ligament (PCL) can be preserved. Following removal of the menisci, cruciate ligaments and posterior osteophytes, the soft tissue balance is checked with a space block and alignment rod (Fig. 6.7). The collateral ligaments should be balanced. If there is any inequality, the proper soft tissue releases should be performed. The release for a residual varus deformity has been well described and it includes a subperiosteal elevation of the deep and superficial medial collateral ligament (MCL). This subperiosteal release of the MCL can be performed with the mini-incision approach, without excessive subcutaneous dissection along the proximal medial tibia. A lateral release for a valgus deformity can be performed through the medial arthrotomy. The "pie crust" technique selectively releases the arcuate ligament, the iliotibial band, and the lateral collateral ligament, with preservation of the popliteus tendon.

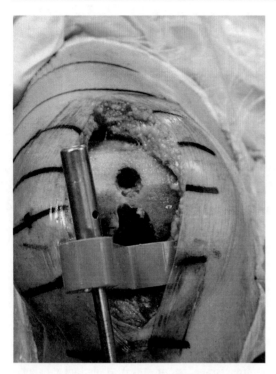

Fig. 6.7 The spacer block determines knee balance and alignment (From Scuderi GR, Tria AJ, Jr., Minimal incision total knee arthroplasty. In: Scuderi GR, Tria AJ, Jr. (eds.), *MIS of the Hip and the Knee*. New York: Springer, 2004, with kind permission of Springer Science + Business Media, Inc.)

Once it is determined that the knee is appropriately balanced, the finishing cuts are performed on both the femur and tibia to allow testing with the provisional components. The knee is flexed to 90° and the bone is resected form the femoral intercondylar notch to accommodate the posterior-stabilized femoral component. To gain exposure to the proximal tibial surface, the knee is hyperflexed and externally rotated. In this position, the femur falls beneath the extensor mechanism and does not interfere with visualization of the proximal tibia. The appropriately sized tibial template is positioned in the correct rotation and the tibia is prepared for the final component.

Patella preparation is performed after femoral and tibial resection. Following removal of the bone from the proximal tibia and distal femur, there is approximately a 20-mm gap, resulting in laxity of the soft tissue envelope, which allows easier manipulation of the patella during preparation. With the knee in either full extension or slight flexion, the patella is tilted. Following measurement of the patella thickness, using the appropriately sized reamer, the patella is resected to the appropriate depth. The three fixation holes are drilled and a trial button placed. The final thickness of the resurfaced patella is measured and compared with the original thickness.

Following all the bone preparation, the trial components are inserted. Since the provisional tibial component is inserted first, the knee is hyperflexed and externally rotated, allowing the tibia to sublux forward through the arthrotomy. After the tibial tray is placed, the knee is then brought back to 90° of flexion, and, with distraction of the joint, the flexion space opens and the provisional femoral component is impacted onto the distal femur. The provisional tibial articular surface is then inserted. If there is difficulty gaining exposure and inserting the tibial articular surface, the knee is placed in mid-flexion, approximately 45–60°, and the articular surface is guided into place. Finally, the trial patellar button is placed. Patellar tracking can be assessed at this time. The incidence of lateral retinacular releases has not been impacted by this limited approach. I have reported a lateral release rate of 15% with both a mini-incision arthrotomy and the standard approach [8]. After the provisional components are tested and thought to result in excellent range of motion, stability, and patellar tracking, they are removed and the bone is prepared for cementation of the final components. The knee is copiously irrigated with pulsatile lavage and dried thoroughly. All patients receive a cemented modular fixed bearing posterior-stabilized knee prosthesis (NexGen LPS-Flex or LPS-Flex Gender Prosthesis, Zimmer, Warsaw, IN). Once the cement is of the appropriate viscosity, the knee is hyperflexed and externally rotated. Cement is placed on the proximal tibia and into the stem hole, and the tibial tray is impacted into place and any excess cement is removed. The knee is brought back to 90° of flexion. Cement is placed along the anterior and distal femur as well as on the posterior condyles of the implant. The femoral component is then impacted in place and all excess cement is

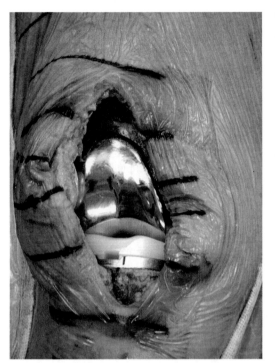

Fig. 6.8 The final components in place (From Scuderi GR, Tria AJ, Jr., Minimal incision total knee arthroplasty. In: Scuderi GR, Tria AJ, Jr. (eds.), *MIS of the Hip and the Knee*. New York: Springer, 2004, with kind permission of Springer Science + Business Media, Inc.)

removed. A careful inspection of the posterior recess and along the margins of the implant should confirm that there is no cement debris. A reduction is performed with a provisional tibial articular surface. The patella is cemented in place and held with the patellar clamp until the cement hardens. The knee is assessed for appropriate balance range of motion, and patellar tracking. If the results are satisfactory, the provisional tibial articular surface is removed and the final tibial polyethylene insert is locked in place. If there is difficulty inserting the final tibial polyethylene component, the knee can be placed in mid-flexion and, with a front-loading tibial tray, the polyethylene insert can be guided into place.

With the final components in place (Fig. 6.8), the tourniquet is released and any bleeding is addressed with electrocautery. The tourniquet is then reinflated for closure and the knee is copiously irrigated with an antibiotic solution.

The arthrotomy is closed over a suction drain in an interrupted fashion using an absorbable suture. The deep tissues and the subcutaneous layer are closed with absorbable sutures and the skin is closed with staples. A light sterile dressing is applied and held in place with a compressive stocking.

Postoperative Management

Following surgery, pain management is achieved with either an indwelling epidural catheter for the first 24 h or a femoral nerve block. This is followed by intravenous patient controlled analgesia (PCA) under the direction of the pain service. Continuous passive motion (CPM) is initiated in the recovery room. Patients begin full weight-bearing ambulation and active range of motion exercises as soon as they are alert, stable, and able to follow the instructions of the physical therapists. Physical therapy is undertaken twice daily. Patients are discharged to either home or a rehabilitation center within 2–4 days depending on their progress with physiotherapy and their social situation. An integrated multidisciplinary postoperative clinical pathway is fundamental to patient satisfaction [9].

Clinical Results

MIS TKA with a limited medial parapatellar arthrotomy is a technique with satisfactory results when the above key steps are followed. In a recently published comparison study [5], the clinical outcome of a group of mini-incision TKA was compared with that of a group of knee arthrotomies performed with a standard approach. The amount of blood reinfused from the postoperative drain was less in the mini-incision group (mean 292 cc) compared with the group of knee arthrotomies performed with a standard approval (mean 683 cc). Postoperative day 3 hemoglobin measurements were similar between the groups. However, the mini-incision group had reduced transfusion requirements. Our current "bloodless surgery" protocol avoids a preoperative anemia by no longer collecting autologous blood preoperatively; checking the preoperative hemoglobin and using erythropoietin when indicated; and using a reinfusion drain in all patients. This protocol has significantly reduced our transfusion rate in unilateral TKA [10].

The average length of hospital stay was similar in the two groups: 3.9 days for patients in the mini-incision group, and 4.2 days for patients in the standard group [5]. Thirty-eight percent of the patients in the mini-incision group were discharged directly to their homes compared with 24% of patients in the standard group. By postoperative day 3, the patients who had mini-incision procedures were walking an average 5.8 m further and climbing 1.2 more stair steps than patients who had standard procedures, but these differences were not significant. On postoperative day 3, the patients who had mini-incision procedures had better flexion than patients who had the standard procedures ($p = 0.014$), with an average 4° of difference. The average postoperative flexion for the mini-incision group on day 3 was 92° (range 48–120°), compared with an average of 88° in the standard arthrotomy group (range 69–105).

While one of the major concerns with the use of MIS TKA is that it will compromise the positioning of components, this has not been our experience. A radiographic analysis has revealed that the average alignment of the prosthesis and the overall limb alignment were consistent with previously published reports [5, 11]. This is most likely due to the fact that the mini-incision approach is a familiar extensile approach permitting adequate visualization in the carefully selected patient without compromising the surgical accuracy. In addition, the procedure is performed with modified instruments, which are similar to prior instrumentation familiar to the surgeon.

Complications are avoided with meticulous surgical technique, and a review of our early experience has been previously reported [5]. In a group of mini-incision TKA, two patients had superficial erythema of the knee that resolved without sequelae; one patient with a varus deformity developed temporary common peroneal nerve palsy at the level of the proximal fibula, which resolved; and one patient had a traumatic patellar dislocation after a fall 12 weeks postoperatively, requiring a repair of the medial retinaculum. There were no skin or wound complications delaying the healing process. In the standard incision group, two patients had superficial erythema of the knee that resolved, one patient required manipulation under anesthesia at 5 weeks postoperatively, and one patient required arthroscopic lysis of adhesions in conjunction with manipulation at 22 weeks. Presently, the mini-incision approach is being used in the majority of my patients without any untoward effects, because I will gradually extend the skin incision and arthrotomy as needed in an effort to avoid complications.

Discussion

MIS TKA has gained popularity over the last several years and the limited medial parapatellar arthrotomy is part of the continuum of these modified approaches with limited access and visibility. The learning curve is short since the arthroplasty is performed with the same surgical technique using modified and smaller instruments that are more adaptable to the limited operative field. With a gradual shortening of the skin incision and medial parapatellar arthrotomy, a smaller and comfortable operative field will be obtained.

Others have reported a similar clinical experience with this approach. Coon and coworkers recently reported on their experience with MIS TKA using both the MIS mini-incision and the MIS quadriceps-sparing techniques [3]. They found a significantly shorter length of stay of 3.4 days versus 5.9 days for the traditional approach. Patients who had MIS had a lower transfusion requirement of 4% versus 34%. Looking at the early functional outcome, MIS patients walked three times farther on the third postoperative day (176 ft versus 58 ft) and had a better range of motion. This study also reported a potential cost reduction to the healthcare system as surgeons performing MIS improve their operative efficiency and further reduce the hospital length of stay.

The definition of success with MIS TKA is dependent upon the expectations of the surgeon, patient, and family. Patients have overwhelmingly become interested in the concept of MIS because of the anticipation of lower morbidity and a more rapid recovery. However, they need to realize that the clinical outcome is not solely dependent on the length of the incision. During preoperative counseling, patients are informed that they will receive the smallest incision possible to allow for proper placement of the prosthesis rather than guaranteed an incision of a specific length. Success is also multifactorial and dependent on appropriate blood loss management, effective pain control, a comprehensive physiotherapy program, and a supportive social services network.

Optimizing patient selection and paying specific attention to the operative details will ensure clinical success. Experience has demonstrated that there are certain patient characteristics that are better suited for MIS TKA. A shorter, thinner female patient with a lower BMI, a narrower femur, and better preoperative range of motion is better suited for MIS. Caution needs to be taken with patients who have rheumatoid arthritis or inflammatory arthritis, limited range of motion with severe fixed angular deformity, or prior surgery. Regarding the surgical technique, it is important to pay attention to the intraoperative details. The surgical procedure has not essentially changed from the standard techniques. The real difference is that the procedure is performed in an operative field with limited visibility. The addition of modified and smaller instruments has made it easier to access the joint with little or no damage to the extensor mechanism. Training of the surgical assistants to position the knee and retractors for specific surgical steps will greatly facilitate the operation. Finally, MIS TKA can easily be converted to a more extensile approach if there is any difficulty with exposure or positioning the instrumentation or the implants during the arthroplasty. TKA is historically a successful operation and the MIS technique should not compromise the outcome.

References

1. Scuderi GR, Tenholder M, Capeci C. Surgical approaches in mini-incision total knee arthroplasty. Clin Orthop Relat Res 428:61–67, 2004
2. Bonutti PM, Neal DJ, Kester MA. Minimal incision total knee arthroplasty using the suspended leg technique. Orthopedics 26:899–903, 2003
3. Coon TM, Tria AJ, Lavernia C, Randall L. The economics of minimally invasive total knee surgery. Semin Arthroplasty 16:235–238, 2005
4. Laskin RS. New techniques and concepts in total knee replacement. Clin Orthop Relat Res 416:151–153, 2003
5. Tenholder M, Clarke HD, Scuderi GR. Minimal incision total knee arthroplasty: the early clinical experience. Clin Orthop Relat Res 440:67–76, 2005
6. Scuderi GR. Minimally invasive total knee arthroplasty. Am J Orthop 7 S:7–11, 2006
7. Kim R, Scuderi GR, Cushner F, et al. Use of lidocaine with epinephrine injection to reduce blood loss in MIS TKA. Proceedings of the 2007 Annual AAOS Meeting, San Diego, CA
8. Cook JL, Scuderi GR, Tenholder M. Incidence of lateral release in total knee arthroplasty in standard and mini approaches. Clin Orthop Relat Res 452:123–126, 2006
9. Scuderi GR. Pre-operative planning and peri-operative management for minimally invasive total knee arthroplasty. Am J Orthopedics 7 S:4–6, 2006
10. Cushner FD, Lee GC, Scuderi GR, et al. Blood loss management in high risk patients undergoing total knee arthroplasty. J Knee Surg 19:249–253, 2006
11. Brassard MF, Insall JN, Scuderi GR, Colizza W. Does modularity affect clinical success? A comparison with a minimum 10-year follow-up. Clin Orthop Relat Res 388:26–32, 2001

MIS TKA with a Subvastus Approach

Mark W. Pagnano

Performing minimally invasive (MIS) total knee arthroplasty (TKA) through a subvastus approach makes sense on an anatomic basis, on a scientific basis, and on a practical basis. Anatomically, the subvastus approach is the only approach that saves the entire quadriceps tendon insertion on the patella [1–5] (Fig. 7.1). Scientifically, the subvastus approach has been shown, in prospective randomized clinical trials, to be superior to the standard medial parapatellar arthrotomy and to the so-called quadriceps-sparing arthrotomy [3, 6, 7] (Table 7.1). Practically, MIS TKA with a subvastus approach is reliable, reproducible, and efficient and allows the MIS technique to be applied to a broad group of patients, not just a highly selected subgroup [8] (Table 7.2).

It is now accepted widely that the tenets of MIS TKA include a smaller skin incision, no eversion of the patella, minimal disruption of the suprapatellar pouch, and minimal disruption of the quadriceps tendon. To what degree any one of those factors contribute to improvements in postoperative function remains unclear. Our initial attempts at MIS TKA using the short medial arthrotomy (sometimes referred to as the quadriceps-sparing approach) and the mini-midvastus splitting approaches were frustrated by some substantial technical difficulties. We then modified the sub-

M.W. Pagnano (✉)
Department of Orthopaedic Surgery,
Mayo Clinic College of Medicine, Mayo Clinic,
Rochester, MN, USA
e-mail: pagnano.mark@mayo.edu

vastus approach to the knee to meet the tenets of MIS TKA and found that it markedly facilitated MIS surgery and allowed MIS surgery to be applied to a broader group of patients. When coupled with instruments designed specifically for small-incision surgery, the modified subvastus approach is reliable, reproducible, and safe. Using a simple set of retractors, this procedure can be done without making any blind cuts or free-hand cuts, and that enhances surgical accuracy and patient safety.

Surgical Technique

The incision starts at the superior pole of the patella, ends at the top of the tibial tubercle, and typically measures 3.5 in. (8.8 cm) in extension. Surgeons should start with a traditional 6- to 8-in. incision and then shorten the incision length over time. The medial skin flap is elevated to clearly delineate the inferior border of the vastus medialis obliquus muscle (VMO). The fascia overlying the VMO is left intact because this helps maintain the integrity of the muscle belly itself throughout the case. The anatomy in this region is very consistent. The inferior edge of the VMO is always found more inferior and more medial than most surgeons anticipate. The muscle fibers of the VMO are oriented at a 50° angle and the VMO tendon always attaches to the midpole of the patella. It is very important to save this edge of tendon from the edge of muscle down to the midpole of the patella. That is where the retractor will rest so that the VMO muscle itself is protected

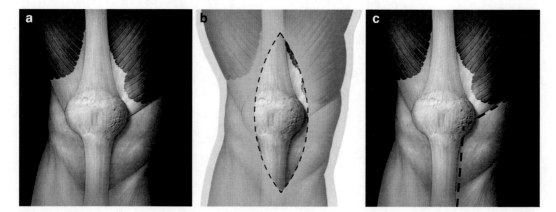

Fig. 7.1 Anatomy of the extensor mechanism. (**a**) The vastus medialis obliquus (VMO) tendon consistently inserts at the midpole of the patella at a 50° angle relative to the long axis of the femur. (**b**) When looking through a surgical incision, one could easily misidentify the most prominent part of the VMO (the point closest to the patella, akin to the bow of the ship) as the most inferior part of the VMO. Because that most prominent portion often lies close to the superior pole of the patella, some surgeons might then mistakenly presume that the VMO inserts at the superior pole of the patella. Additional medial dissection will delineate the inferior border of the VMO, which is more inferior and more medial than most surgeons anticipate. (**c**) The arthrotomy for the subvastus exposure parallels the inferior border of the VMO, intersects the patella at the midpole, and then is turned straight distally to parallel the medial margin of the patellar tendon (Copyright Mayo Foundation, used with permission)

Table 7.1 Prospective randomized trials of the subvastus approach in total knee arthroplasty

Authors	No. of patients randomized	Study variable	Key findings
Roysam and Oakley [7]	89	Subvastus versus medial parapatellar approach	1. Subvastus had earlier straight medial parapatellar leg raising; $p < 0.001$ 2. Subvastus used fewer narcotics week 1; $p < 0.001$ 3. Subvastus had greater knee flexion at 1 week; $p < 0.001$
Aglietti et al. [6]	60	Subvastus versus Zimmer quadriceps-sparing approach	1. Subvastus had earlier straight leg raising; $p = 0.004$ 2. Subvastus had better flexion at 10 days $p = 0.01$ 3. Subvastus had better flexion at 30 days; $p = 0.03$
Faure et al. [3]	20	Subvastus versus medial parapatellar approach	1. Subvastus had greater strength at 1 week and 1 month 2. Subvastus had fewer lateral releases done 3. Subvastus was preferred by patients 4:1

Table 7.2 Clinical results with the minimally invasive subvastus approach in 103 consecutive patients with osteoarthritis

Sex	Age (range)	Weight (range)	Operative time (range)	Functional outcomes mean
61 women; 42 men	66 years (40–90 years)	198 lbs (137–305 lbs)	58 min (35–115 min)	1. Hospital stay: 2.8 days 2. Normal daily activities: 7 days 3. No walker: 14 days 4. No cane: 21 days 5. Drive: 28 days 6. Walk ½ mile: 42 days 7. Flexion at 8 weeks: 116°

From Pagnano et al. [8]

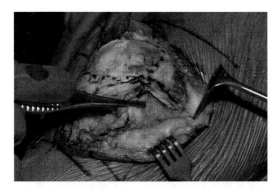

Fig. 7.2 The arthrotomy starts medially along the inferior border of the VMO and extends to the midpole of the patella at the same 50° angle as the muscle fibers of the VMO

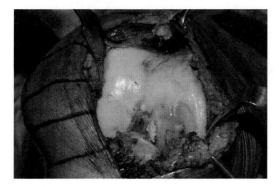

Fig. 7.3 With surprisingly little force, the patella is retracted completely into the lateral gutter. The knee is then flexed to 90° providing exposure of both condyles of the distal femur

throughout the case. The arthrotomy is made along the inferior edge of the VMO down to the midpole of the patella (do not be tempted to cheat this superiorly, because that will hinder, not help, the ultimate exposure) (Fig. 7.2). The proximal limb of the arthrotomy parallels the inferior edge of the VMO and is made at the same 50° angle relative to the long axis of the femur. At the midpole of the patella, the arthrotomy is directed straight distally along the medial border of the patellar tendon. A 90° bent-Hohmann retractor is placed in the lateral gutter and rests against the robust edge of VMO tendon that was preserved during the exposure. Surprisingly little force is needed to completely retract the patella into the lateral gutter. Any substantial medial or inferior osteophytes on the patella are debrided with a

rongeur. The knee is then flexed to 90°, providing good exposure of both distal femoral condyles (Fig. 7.3). If the patella does not slide easily into the lateral gutter, typically it is because a portion of the medial patellofemoral ligament remains attached to the patella. That occurs if the proximal limb of the arthrotomy is made in too horizontal a fashion rather than at the 50° angle that parallels the VMO. By releasing that tight band of tissue, the patella will translate laterally without substantial difficulty.

The distal femur is cut with a modified intramedullary resection guide. Bringing the knee out to 60° of flexion better exposes the anterior portion of the distal femur. When a very small skin incision is used, the distal femur is cut one condyle at a time with the intramedullary portion of the cutting guide left in place for added stability. If a slightly longer skin incision is used, the distal cutting guide can be pinned in place and both condyles cut in a standard fashion.

The proximal tibia is cut next and, by doing that, more room is made for subsequently sizing and rotating the femoral component (the most difficult part of any MIS TKA). Three retractors are placed precisely to get good exposure of the entire surface of the tibia: a pickle-fork retractor posteriorly provides an anterior drawer and protects the neurovascular structures; and bent-Hohmann retractors medially and laterally protect the collateral ligaments and define the perimeter of the tibial bone (Fig. 7.4). The tibial resection is done with an extramedullary guide optimized for small incision surgery. The tibia is cut in one piece using a narrow but thick saw blade that fits the captured guide. The narrow blade is more maneuverable in the smaller guide and provides better tactile feedback for the surgeon to detect when the posterior and lateral tibial cortices have been cut.

The femoral sizing and rotation guide is thin enough to be pinned to the distal femur and then the knee can be brought out to 60° of flexion to visualize the anterior femur for accurate sizing (Fig. 7.5). At 60° of flexion, a retractor is placed anteriorly and the surgeon can see under direct vision that the femoral cortex will not be notched. Clearing some of the synovium overlying the

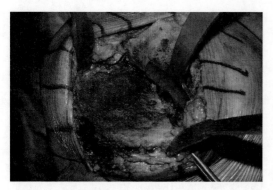

Fig. 7.4 After the distal femur has been cut, the tibia is prepared next, and that is done to provide more working room for subsequently sizing and rotating the femoral component (the most difficult part of any MIS TKA). Good exposure of the entire surface of the tibia is accomplished with three retractors placed precisely: a pickle-fork retractor posteriorly to provide an anterior drawer, and bent-Hohmann retractors medially and laterally to protect the collateral ligaments and define the perimeter of the tibial bone

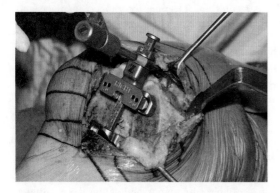

Fig. 7.5 The femoral sizing and rotation guide is designed to be pinned to the distal femur and is thin enough that the knee can subsequently be brought out to 60° of flexion to visualize the anterior femur for accurate sizing

anterior femoral cortex helps ensure that femoral sizing is accurate. The femoral finishing guide is adjusted medially or laterally. Femoral rotation is confirmed by referencing the surgeon's choice of the posterior condyles, Whiteside's line, or the transepicondylar axis, each of which can be defined with this subvastus approach. After the femoral and tibial cuts are made, the surgeon can carry out final ligament releases and check flexion and extension gap balance in whatever fashion is desired.

Patellar preparation with this surgical approach is left until the end. Cutting the patella is not required for exposure and, by preparing the patella last, the risk of inadvertent damage to the cut surface of the patella is minimized. The patella cut is done freehand or with the surgeon's choice of cutting or reaming guides. When a patellar cutting guide is used, the trial components are removed because then the entire limb can shorten, taking tension off the extensor mechanism and allowing easier access to the patella for preparation.

The modular tibial tray is cemented first, then the femur, and finally the patella. The tibia is subluxed forward with the aid of the pickle-fork retractor and the medial and lateral margins of the tibia are exposed well with 90° bent-Hohmann retractors. Care is taken to remove excess cement from around the tibial base plate, particularly posterolaterally. The femur is exposed for cementing by placing bent-Hohmann retractors on the medial and lateral sides proximal to the collateral ligament insertions on the femur. A third retractor is placed under the VMO, where it overlies the anterior femur. Cement is applied to the entire undersurface of femoral implant prior to impaction. Special attention is paid to removing excess cement from the distal lateral surface of the femur because this area is difficult to see after the patella is cemented in place (Fig. 7.6). At this point, the real tibial insert can be placed or a trial insert can be used at the surgeon's discretion. The patella is cemented last. After the cement has hardened, the knee is put through a range of motion and final balancing and patellar tracking are assessed (Fig. 7.7).

The tourniquet is deflated so that any small bleeders in the subvastus space can be identified and coagulated. The closure of the arthrotomy starts by reapproximating the corner of capsule to the extensor mechanism at the midpole of the patella. Then three interrupted zero-Vicryl sutures are placed along the proximal limb of the arthrotomy (Fig. 7.8). These sutures can usually be placed deep to the VMO muscle itself and

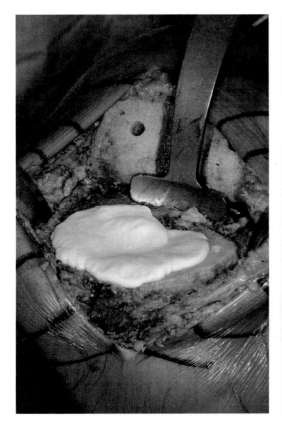

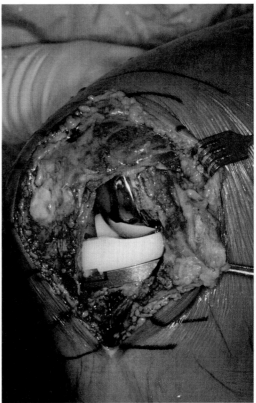

Fig. 7.6 Modular tibial components facilitate the cementing process and it is easiest to cement the tibia first. Excess cement is carefully removed, with particular attention given to the posterolateral corner of the knee

Fig. 7.7 With the final components in place, patellar tracking and range of motion are assessed

grasp either fibrous tissue or the synovium attached to the distal or undersurface of the VMO instead of the muscle itself. These first four sutures are most easily placed with the knee in extension but are then tied with the knee at 90° of flexion to avoid overtightening the medial side and creating an iatrogenic patella baja postoperatively. A deep drain is placed in the knee joint and the distal/vertical limb of the arthrotomy is closed with multiple interrupted zero-Vicryl sutures placed with the knee in 90° of flexion. The skin is closed in layers. Staples are used, not a subcuticular suture. More tension is routinely placed on the skin during MIS TKA surgery than in standard open surgery, and our experience suggests the potential for wound-healing problems is magnified if the skin

is handled multiple times as is the case with a running subcuticular closure.

Discussion

Minimally invasive total knee arthroplasty with a subvastus approach has proved reliable, reproducible, and efficient. The technique is amenable to stepwise surgeon learning and can be applied to a substantial range of patients who require total knee arthroplasty not just a selected subgroup. There are patients who are not good candidates for any MIS TKA procedure, including those with marked knee stiffness, fragile skin, or marked obesity. Similarly, any knee with patella baja will be markedly difficult with an MIS approach because subluxing the patella laterally often is not possible. In those cases, a

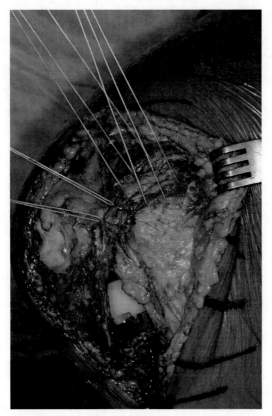

after MIS TKA. Maximizing the early gains after surgery (minimal pain, early ambulation, rapid hospital discharge) typically requires a combination of advanced anesthetic techniques, a multimodal pain management program, a rapid rehabilitation protocol, and appropriate patient expectations. How much each of those contributes versus how much the surgical technique contributes to early functional improvement has not been determined scientifically.

References

1. Pagnano MW, Meneghini RM, Trousdale RT. Anatomy of the extensor mechanism in reference to quadriceps-sparing TKA. Clin Orthop Relat Res 2006 Nov, (452):102–105
2. Chang CH, Chen KH, Yang RS, Liu TK. Muscle torques in total knee arthroplasty with subvastus and parapatellar approaches. Clin Orthop Relat Res 2002, 398:189–195
3. Faure BT, Benjamin JB, Lindsey B, Volz RG, Schutte D. Comparison of the subvastus and paramedian surgical approaches in bilateral knee arthroplasty. J Arthroplasty 1993, 8(5):511–516
4. Gore DR, Sellinger DS, Gassner KJ, Glaeser ST. Subvastus approach for total knee arthroplasty. Orthopedics 2003, 26:33–35
5. Hoffman AA, Plaster RL, Murdock LE. Subvastus (southern) approach for primary total knee arthroplasty. Clin Orthop Relat Res 1991, 269:70–77
6. Aglietti P, Baldini A. A prospective, randomized study of the mini subvastus versus quad-sparing approaches for TKA. Presented at the Interim Meeting of the Knee Society. September 8, 2005, New York, NY
7. Roysam GS, Oakley MJ. Subvastus approach for total knee arthroplasty: a prospective, randomized, and observer-blinded trial. J Arthroplasty 2001, 16:454–457
8. Pagnano MW, Leone JM, Hanssen AD, Lewallen DG. Minimally invasive total knee arthroplasty with an optimized subvastus approach: a consecutive series of 103 patients. Presented at American Academy of Orthopaedic Surgeons Annual Meeting. 2005, Washington DC

Fig. 7.8 The tourniquet should be let down and any small bleeders in the subvastus space should be cauterized. The closure is done by first reapproximating the corner of capsule at the midpole of the patella. Then three interrupted sutures are placed through the deep layer of synovium to close the knee joint itself. Those four sutures are tied with the knee at 90° of flexion to avoid creating iatrogenic patella baja

traditional skin incision and more extensile exposure are in the interest of patient and surgeon alike.

Surgeons should be aware that changes in surgical technique alone are unlikely to provide the dramatic early improvements in postoperative function that some surgeons have described

Mini-midvastus Total Knee Arthroplasty

8

Steven B. Haas, Samuel J. Macdessi, and Mary Ann Manitta

Total knee arthroplasty (TKA) is now considered a gold-standard treatment of advanced arthritis of the knee [1–4]. The early convalescence with standard surgical techniques however is longer than that of total hip arthroplasty, with significant pain and disability from the surgical insult delaying functional recovery. The traditional surgical approach for exposure in knee replacement remains the median parapatellar (MPP) approach. This was initially described by von Langenbeck in 1874 and then popularized by Insall in 1971 [5]. Although this approach is the only true extensile approach, it incises the quadriceps tendon, which may delay functional recovery.

Both the midvastus [6] and subvastus [7] approaches have been described to minimize this trauma. The subvastus approach does not violate any portion of the vastus medialis obliquus (VMO) tendon, whereas the midvastus approach incises a small portion of this tendon, usually up to the superior pole of the patella. Technically, it is more difficult to expose the distal femur through the subvastus approach as preservation of the quadriceps attachment reduces proximal surgical visualization.

The midvastus approach is a compromise between the excellent exposure afforded by the MPP approach and the advantages provided by the subvastus approach. With this in mind, the authors developed a minimally invasive (MIS) TKA technique using a modification of the midvastus approach and have entitled it the "mini-midvastus approach." The fundamental principles of this technique are blunt and minimal splitting of the VMO, avoidance of patellar eversion, minimization of soft tissue violation, adequate visualization through the mobile window, and the use of smaller instrumentation. By adhering to these principles, we think that early patient recovery can be optimized without compromising the factors that contribute to long-term success.

Midvastus Approach

The midvastus approach was popularized by Engh [6, 8] in an attempt to minimize violation of the quadriceps mechanism. It was thought that this approach would enhance patellofemoral stability, increase postoperative quadriceps control, and decrease scarring in the quadriceps mechanism should revision surgery be required.

The midvastus approach has been studied in several randomized trials comparing it with the

S.B. Haas (✉)
Weill Medical College of Cornell University,
New York, NY, USA
e-mail: haass@hss.edu

Department of Orthopedic Surgery,
Hospital for Special Surgery, New York, NY, USA

S.J. Macdessi
Sydney Knee Specialists, Edgecliff, Australia

M.A. Manitta
Department of Orthopedics, Hospital for Special Surgery,
New York, NY, USA

MPP approach. Dalury and Jiranek [9] noted greater quadriceps strength at 6 weeks and earlier return of straight leg raise in a bilateral knee replacement study of 100 patients. In a similar but larger study of 100 patients, White et al. [10] also noted less pain at 8 days and 6 weeks in the midvastus group, a greater ability to straight leg raise at 8 days, and less patellar retinacular releases. Unilateral randomized trials have also verified these results. Maestro et al. [11] found a higher incidence of lateral release, loss of knee extension, and reduced range of motion with the MPP approach. Bathis et al. [12] reported early improvements in pain, early quadriceps strength, and proprioception with the midvastus approach. Parentis et al. [13] noted a trend for increased early functional recovery and significantly less blood loss in patients who had undergone a midvastus approach. Engh in 1997 found no difference in functional recovery, range of motion, or radiographic parameters in either group. Likewise, Keating et al. [14] found no difference in early functional recovery.

The midvastus approach may also influence patellar tracking by minimizing the amount of detachment of the VMO from the medial patella. This may decrease the need to perform a lateral release, which can increase postoperative morbidity, with increased lateral swelling and pain. Engh et al. [15] reported a lateral release rate of 3% in patients undergoing a midvastus approach compared with 50% using the MPP approach. White et al. [10] noted a 13% rate in the MPP approach compared with 8% in the midvastus approach which was statistically significant. Additionally, both Maestro et al. [11] and Parentis et al. [13] noted fewer lateral releases. Keating et al. [14] noted no differences in lateral release rates.

Very little has been reported on postoperative patellar positioning using the midvastus approach. Ozkoc et al. [16] assessed time-dependent changes in patellar tracking in a randomized trial comparing the midvastus with the MPP approach. Although early tilt angles were similar, late patellar tilt was noted in the MPP group. Both early and late lateral subluxation and worse congruence angles were noted in the MPP group.

Anatomical Considerations with the Midvastus Approach

Cooper et al. [17] performed a cadaveric study assessing the neurovascular relationships in the midvastus approach. The perforating vessels were on average 8.8 cm from the patella. They recommend a safe distance for sharp muscle splitting to be 4.5 cm. If further exposure is necessary, the remaining muscle fibers can then be bluntly split to the level of the vastoadductor membrane and adductor magnus tendon without neurovascular injury.

Theoretically, concern exists of denervation of the distal portion of the VMO with the midvastus approach. Cooper et al. [17] noted extensive branching of the femoral nerve en route to the oblique portion of the muscle. Using the midvastus approach, the distal muscle segment could only be denervated by splitting the muscle fibers to the point of attachment to the vastoadductor membrane because the femoral nerve lies in a fascial tunnel just deep to this point.

Parentis et al. [13] found a 43% incidence of early VMO denervation on electromyographic testing when using the midvastus approach with the patella everted. They compared this with the MPP approach and found no muscle denervation changes in this group. A muscle split of approximately 10–15 cm was employed. Four of six cases with acute changes were distal to the muscle split. In patients with chronic changes, once again, five of six were in the distal portion of the muscle. One patient had acute and chronic changes both proximally and distally. Theoretically, patellar subluxation with greater stretch on the quadriceps mechanism may increase the risk of neuropraxia. Despite these electromyographic changes, there was a trend for superior functional recovery for up to 6 weeks in the midvastus group.

In a 5-year follow-up study of the same patient group, Kelly et al. [18] found that only two of the nine patients had persistent chronic abnormalities, with one having reinnervation changes and the other demonstrating ongoing denervation. Both of these cases were distal to the muscle split and both were performed by sharp dissection. All patients who had the muscle split performed bluntly had a normal electromyographic study. This raises the possibility of direct trauma to the nerve. No functional deficits were observed.

We recently performed a comparative study of 20 consecutive patients who had undergone a MIS-TKA using a midvastus approach without patellar eversion [19]. Electromyographic analysis of the vastus medialis muscle above and below the muscle split was performed. Average time from surgery to electromyographic analysis was 3.9 months. Four patients (20%) demonstrated mildly abnormal polyphasic changes consistent with mild denervation only. Two were distal and two were proximal to the muscle split. At a similar follow-up interval, this was considerably less than that noted by Parentis et al. where the patella was everted.

The Mini-midvastus Modification

In 2001, the senior author (SBH) developed a modification to the midvastus approach where the patella is subluxed and not everted. This has been termed the mini-midvastus approach. Theoretically, this places less stress on the extensor mechanism, thereby minimizing the length of the muscle split required. By using the principles of the mobile window, downsized anatomically shaped instruments, and minimizing tibial subluxation, less splitting of the muscle is required.

Another potential advantage of the mini-midvastus approach is the need for smaller incisions. The incision with the traditional medial parapatellar approach is generally carried proximally to the end of the split in the quadriceps tendon. This is not necessary with the mini-midvastus technique. In fact, we have found that with improvements in instrumentation, a TKA can be safely and accurately performed through an 8.5–12 cm skin incision (Fig. 8.1).

Preoperative Assessment

Several points are pertinent in the assessment of a potential candidate for MIS-TKA. Clinical

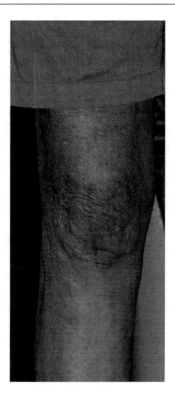

Fig. 8.1 Appearance of smaller incision used in MIS total knee replacement (TKR)

examination should focus on the patient's size, knee range of motion, presence of scars, deformity of the extremity, and the limb's neurovascular status. Radiographs are interpreted for deformity, bone loss, presence of patellar baja and overall bone quality. All patients undergo a complete medical evaluation prior to their arthroplasty.

Although no absolute contraindications exist, certain patients are more amenable to undergo a MIS-TKA. Approximately 75% of patients have this approach whereas the remainder have a limited MPP approach performed with an identical technique. Relative contraindications include men with a substantial quadriceps muscle mass, significant obesity (body mass index [BMI] greater than 40) and the presence of severe coronal plane deformity. We also do not use a MIS-TKA technique with flexion contractures of more than 25°, passive flexion of less than 80°, or in patients with severe patellar baja or significant scarring of the quadriceps mechanism.

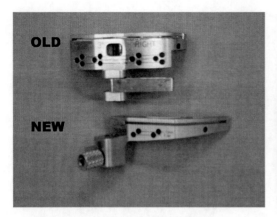

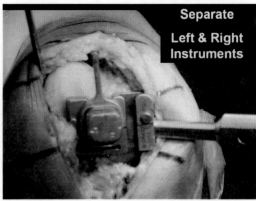

Fig. 8.2 *Top* – Standard Genesis II Tibial Cutting Block. *Bottom* – MIS Genesis II Tibial Cutting Block (Smith and Nephew)

Fig. 8.3 Preparing a femur with a right-sided MIS valgus/rotation guide. The stylus is aligned with the AP axis line (Whiteside's line)

Instrumentation

Specialized instrumentation is critical in performing this procedure. Most systems today have made appropriate instrument modifications for a MIS-TKA to be performed. We use the Genesis II (Smith and Nephew, Memphis, TN) High-Flex posterior-stabilized or Journey (Smith and Nephew) systems.

To meet the demands of a mini-midvastus approach, cutting blocks and guides were made smaller with rounded edges to be accommodated through smaller incisions. Additionally, side-specific instruments have been developed so that the extensor mechanism does not impede placement of cutting blocks (Fig. 8.2). We also use a saw blade that is rigid with a narrow body that fans out at the distal tip to facilitate bone cuts.

The tibial guide has a side-specific medial wing that hugs the medial tibial plateau. The lateral wing was removed because it was impeded by the position of the patellar ligament. The lateral portion was never used to cut through, because iatrogenic laceration of the patellar ligament may result. This modification allows the lateral plateau to be cut from both anterior to posterior and medial to lateral.

Femoral instruments include a side-specific valgus alignment system in which the bulk of the guide can be placed medially where there is ample exposure (Fig. 8.3). The anterior femoral cutting guide, distal femoral cutting block, and the four-in-one finishing are narrower in the medial to lateral dimension and permit more freely angled cuts. The remainder of the instruments, including the anterior resection stylus, the distal resection stylus, the housing resection block (for posterior-stabilized knees), and femoral sizing guide, have been downsized. Additionally, the anterior stylus is angled to allow placement under the skin when referencing the preliminary anterior cut.

Surgical Technique

Anesthesia

All patients receive epidural anesthesia, which is continued for 48 h. Patients also receive a Marcaine femoral nerve block, which we have found aids significantly in postoperative pain control. Intravenous cephazolin is our antibiotic of choice. Patients with significant allergies to penicillins are administered vancomycin.

Patient Set-up

An above-knee tourniquet is applied, with protection of the skin by wool. A sandbag is placed under the drapes at the level of the opposite ankle so that the knee can sit flexed at approximately 70–90°. The majority of the procedure is done in this position. Hyperflexion is sometimes required to prepare the proximal tibia and insert the definitive tibial tray. A lateral support is used so that the leg sits without being held by an assistant.

Exposure

Landmarks for the skin incision are the borders of the patella and the tibial tubercle. These are marked and then a longitudinal incision line is drawn at the junction of the middle and medial thirds of the patella. The incision extends from 1 cm above the superior pole of the patella to the proximal half of the tibial tubercle on its medial side. Our typical skin incision length is between 8.5 and 12 cm. However, we have no hesitation to extend this at any stage if there appears to be undue tension, especially at the distal apex of the incision.

A medial arthrotomy is performed. This extends from the superior pole of the patella to the level of the tibial tubercle. We leave a 5-mm cuff of tissue adjacent to the tubercle to aid in closure later on. The VMO is identified and an oblique split is made in the muscle in the line of its fibers at the level of the superior pole of the patella.

The first centimeter of the muscle split is started sharply but the remainder is performed bluntly with a finger, gently separating the muscle fibers. Performing the split completely by sharp dissection risks damaging the distal innervation of the vastus musculature. The muscle split generally is between 2 and 3 cm in length. The suprapatellar pouch is preserved except in cases of severe inflammatory disease.

With the knee extended, a subperiosteal dissection is carried around the medial pretibial border, releasing the meniscotibial attachments. The patella is then retracted laterally and a partial excision of the infrapatellar fat pad is performed. We also excise the medial fat pad at this stage. The tibial attachments of the anterior cruciate ligament and the anterior horn of the lateral meniscus are released. This allows placement of a thin bent Hohmann retractor laterally to sublux the patella. A small synovial window is made over the anterolateral femoral cortex to aid in our initial anterior femoral resection.

This is found more commonly in men and sometimes require initial patellar resection to assist in patellar subluxation. We caution against initial patellar resection in older, osteoporotic females because of the risk of iatrogenic crushing of the patellar bone during lateral retraction.

Femoral Preparation

Femoral preparation is performed first to relax the extension space. This is done with the knee in 70° of flexion. Limiting knee flexion places the soft tissue window over the distal and anterior femur. Hyperflexion must be avoided because it not only tightens the extensor mechanism but also limits exposure. A thin, bent Hohmann retractor is placed laterally around the margin of the femoral condyle without excessive lateral traction to hold the patella subluxed.

The anteroposterior axis (Whiteside's line) is marked on the distal femur and is used as the major landmark for establishing component rotation. The posterior condylar axis is used as a secondary reference in varus knees, where it is most reproducible. The transepicondylar axis is more difficult to assess because it requires excessive retraction of the patella laterally.

A 9.5-mm drill is used to enter the femoral canal at a starting point in the notch just anterior to the posterior cruciate ligament insertion on the femur. The canal is then suctioned of its marrow contents to reduce fat embolization risk. An intramedullary alignment guide set at 5° of valgus relative to the anatomic axis is inserted. We only use posterior paddles for additional referencing if there is concern about rotational alignment. An anteroposterior (AP) stylus guide inserted over the rod is placed in line with the marking of the AP axis, and the block is pinned in place. An anterior referencing guide is then slid under the quadriceps mechanism touching the anterolateral femoral cortex, which usually represents the highest point.

The preliminary anterior resection guide is then pinned in place, and the preliminary cut is performed. We prefer to use an anterior resection first technique, so that later corrections in rotational or sagittal placement can be made if we are not satisfied with our initial position. Along with this, this cut relaxes the extensor mechanism prior to placement of the distal cutting guide and allows the guide to sit more evenly on a flat surface.

We then perform our distal femoral resection. Additional retraction is not required at this point because the guide's wedge shape usually retracts the proximal tissues adequately. The block is secured with two headed pins, the intramedullary rod is removed, and the distal resection is performed.

The femoral component size is then determined. The knee may require further flexion so that the posterior paddles can be passed behind the posterior condyles. If we are between sizes, we prefer to choose the smaller component size so as not to overtighten the flexion space. We then pin the appropriate four-in-one cutting guide in place, and once again assess our rotation. It is critical at this stage that a thin bent Hohmann retractor is placed deep to the medial collateral ligament (MCL) for protection. The femoral resection is performed in the following order: posterior condyles, posterior chamfer, anterior resection, and anterior chamfer.

Tibial Preparation

The proximal tibial resection is then performed (Fig. 8.4). We prefer extramedullary instrumentation however intramedullary rod alignment can be used with this technique. The knee is flexed to approximately 90°. Excessive external rotation, which is often utilized in the standard approach, must be avoided because this decreases visualization of the lateral compartment by rotating the lateral tibial plateau under the femur. A thin bent Hohmann retractor is then placed medially and laterally, to once again protect the MCL and the extensor mechanism. Any overhanging anteromedial osteophytes are removed at this stage with a rongeur so that the tibial resection guide can sit

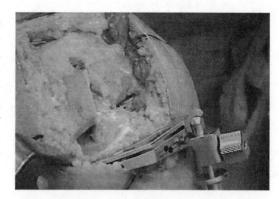

Fig. 8.4 Preparing a tibia with a MIS tibial cutting block (From Haas SB, Lehman AP, Manitta MA. Mini-midvastus total knee arthroplasty. In: Scuderi GR, Tria AJ Jr, Berger RA (eds.), MIS Techniques in Orthopedics, New York, Springer, 2006, with kind permission of Springer Science+Business Media, Inc.)

in direct contact with the margin of the tibia. The tibial guide is placed parallel to the tibial crest proximally. We also use the tibialis anterior tendon over the ankle and the second metatarsal as reference points distally. The posterior slope is then adjusted so that the alignment guide is parallel to the fibular shaft. We aim for an 11-mm resection off the intact side. The guide is then pinned in place. An Aufranc retractor is placed posteriorly in order to protect the posterior neurovascular structures without changing the position of the knee.

We then perform the proximal tibial resection. In order for the blade to be captured by the cutting guide, the saw must initially be angled at 45° aiming posteriorly. Once within the bone, the medial resection can be safely completed directing the blade in an anterior to posterior direction. We then direct the blade laterally to complete the resection. If we are in any doubt of the depth of the resection, we prefer to leave a small rim of bone. It is much safer to remove this later during the procedure as exposure increases, than to aim to remove the bone in one piece and cause an iatrogenic injury to the ligaments or, less commonly, the neurovascular bundle. The alignment of our tibial cut is then rechecked using an alignment rod connected to a spacer block.

The knee is then placed in 90° of flexion. Using laminar spreaders, we assess the posterior

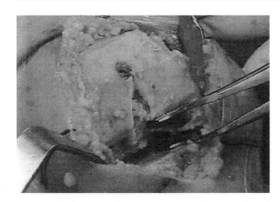

Fig. 8.5 A laminar spreader is placed after bone resection. Good visualization for resection of the meniscus and posterior cruciate ligament (PCL) and for posterior osteophyte removal (From Haas SB, Lehman AP, Manitta MA. Mini-midvastus total knee arthroplasty. In: Scuderi GR, Tria AJ Jr, Berger RA (eds.), MIS Techniques in Orthopedics, New York, Springer, 2006, with kind permission of Springer Science + Business Media, Inc.)

condyles for any retained osteophytes (Fig. 8.5). These are removed with a curved osteotome and aid in reestablishing flexion capability. The meniscal remnants are excised at this stage along with the posterior cruciate ligament (if a posterior stabilized system is being used). We then place spacer blocks into both the flexion and extension spaces to ensure that we have obtained symmetrical spaces with adequate resection levels. Additionally, it is a useful tool to predict later soft tissue releases.

The knee is then flexed to 90–120° and an Aufranc retractor is once again placed posteriorly. This is the only time prior to component insertion that hyperflexion may be necessary. An appropriately sized tibial component is then pinned in place with one pin on the medial side. The proximal tibia is then reamed and broached to accept the definitive prosthesis. We then remove any overhanging tibial osteophytes, which are most commonly found posteromedially.

Final Preparation

Once we have confirmed that no further bone resection is required, we complete our femoral preparation. We place the posterior stabilized box cutter in place and mark the outline with a marking pen by drawing lines on the inner side of the resection box. We temporarily remove it to ensure adequate mediolateral positioning. We have found that lining up the inside of the cutting box with the inner margin of the medial femoral condyle is a useful tool with this prosthesis. Overall, we aim for slight lateral position to optimize patellar tracking. Medial overhang should be avoided, because this is a cause of capsular pain. The guide is then pinned in place and the box is prepared.

If the patella is being resurfaced, it is usually done at this stage. It is easier to wait until both femoral and tibial cuts have been performed as the reduced tension on the extensor mechanism allows the patella to be more easily averted. The patella is then prepared for a trial component. Once the trial is in place, we chamfer the lateral margin with a saw to minimize lateral retinacular impingement.

The trial femoral component is then inserted. We then perform a trial reduction with a variety of inserts and assess for coronal plane stability with the knee in both extension and at 90° of flexion. Soft tissue releases are then performed until satisfactory balance is achieved. Patellofemoral tracking is then observed. If this is found to be suboptimal, it is rechecked with the tourniquet deflated to ensure that a lateral retinacular release is not required.

Component Insertion

We prefer the use of cemented implants; however, noncemented devices may be used. Prior to cementing, the bone surfaces are lavaged under pulsatile pressure to achieve a bloodless and dry bone bed. A bone plug is fashioned and impacted into the femoral hole of the intercondylar notch. Occasionally, sclerotic bone requires drilling with a 2.5-mm drill to enhance cement interdigitation.

The tibial component is inserted first. Exposure is obtained using an identical technique to that employed when inserting the trial component. The posterolateral overhang, which frequently occurs with symmetric tibial implants can lead to difficulty with implant insertion and cement removal. For this reason, we prefer to use an asymmetric tibial base plate to facilitate clearance of the femoral condyle during implantation and subsequent cement removal. Once the tibial component has been implanted, the femoral and patellar components are inserted along with a trial polyethylene insert.

Removal of cement from the posterior margins of the tibia can be aided by placing the knee in extension and applying traction prior to the femoral component implantation. A small curved curette can then be swept posteriorly along the margin of the tibial component to help remove any additional cement. On the femoral side, initial excessive proximal retraction should be avoided to remove cement when the component is being implanted at 90° of flexion. It is best to only remove the cement extruded into the intercondylar notch and the condylar margins at this stage. A trial liner is inserted and the knee is then taken into extension. The mobile window will then easily deliver the anterior femoral cortex into view to remove the remaining extruded cement without the need for retraction.

The patellar component is then placed and clamped and the cement is allowed to harden. Any additional cement is removed at this stage. The definitive polyethylene insert is then inserted. If using a posterior-stabilized insert, the surgeon should begin insertion of the polyethylene in 90° of flexion. The knee should then be brought into extension to engage the locking mechanism. The poly liner is locked with the knee in 5–15° of flexion.

Closure

The tourniquet is deflated at this stage and bleeding is controlled. The knee is copiously lavaged with normal saline solution and two drains are inserted. The capsular layer is closed by placing 0-Vicryl sutures in to the VMO tendon and perimuscular fascia. Three to five sutures will usually suffice. The remainder of the arthrotomy and the subcutaneous tissues are closed with interrupted sutures as well. The authors prefer to use 0-Vicryl sutures for the capsular layer and deep fat and 3/0

Vicryl for the subcutaneous layers. Clips are used to oppose the skin edges.

Rehabilitation

All patients are started on a continuous passive motion (CPM) machine in the recovery room and flexion is increased as pain allows. Weight bearing is commenced on the first postoperative day. All patients receive Coumadin for thromboembolic prophylaxis and foot compressive devices are used until the patient is ambulating unassisted. A patient-controlled epidural is continued until the second postoperative day, when it is removed and the patient is placed on oral analgesics.

Results

The senior author (SBH) has performed over 750 MIS-TKAs using the mini-midvastus technique. It is now used in the majority of primary TKAs being performed. Our initial research [20] on this technique involved a comparative study of 40 TKAs performed using a standard technique with 40 MIS-TKAs using the mini-midvastus modification where the patella was subluxed but not everted. There were no preoperative differences in demographics, range of motion, Knee Society Scores, or function scores between the two groups.

Patients achieved return of motion faster in the MIS-TKA group. Mean flexion for the MIS-TKA group at 6 and 12 weeks was 114° (range 90–132°) and 122° (range 103–135°) respectively, compared with 95° (range 65–125°) and 110° (range 80–125°) for the control group. At 1 year, the MIS-TKA group retained higher mean flexion angles of 125° versus 116° in the control group. Knee Society Scores were also higher in the MIS-TKA group. There were no differences in radiographic alignment. Additionally, no infections, extensor mechanisms, or neurovascular complications occurred.

We recently performed a retrospective analysis of 335 consecutive patients (391 knees) who had underwent a MIS-TKA using the mini-midvastus approach from September 2001 to September

2004 [21]. There were 248 women and 87 men. One third of patients had a BMI of between 30 and 39. The mean preoperative range of motion was 109°. The mean postoperative range of motion was 111° at 6 weeks, 121° at 3 months, and 125° at both 1 and 2 years. We observed no increased complication rate with this approach. There were no fractures, extensor mechanism complications, or neurovascular complications. Our infection rate was 0.5%.

Laskin et al. [22] performed a case-matched outcome study in patients undergoing MIS-TKA using a mini-midvastus approach compared with those having had a MPP approach. The surgeries on this occasion differed in that a cruciate-retaining condylar knee (Genesis II, Smith and Nephew) was used. Patients in the MIS-TKA group had lower pain scores and lower average total morphine sulfate usage when compared with the control arm. Mean flexion in the MIS-TKA group was greater at 6 weeks (115° vs. 110°). At 3 months, the groups had equalized with each other. No differences in limb alignment or stability were noted.

Laskin [23] also reviewed 100 consecutive patients undergoing the same MIS-TKA technique with a mean follow-up of 2.4 years. Patients were excluded from this technique if they had flexion of less than 80°, a flexion contracture of greater than 20°, prior open knee surgery, or rheumatoid arthritis. Weight, severity of deformity, or coronal plane instability was not a contraindication to this technique. The mean passive flexion measured 114° at 4 weeks and 122° at 2 years. Only one tibial component was malpositioned in 4° of varus in a man with a BMI of 40. No femoral components were malpositioned. It was concluded that the surgical approach was not applicable to patients with a BMI of greater than 40 or severe fixed valgus deformity.

Conclusion

The mini-midvastus approach appears to aid in early functional recovery with a more rapid return of motion and possibly a greater ultimate range of motion than the MPP approach. The mini-midvastus approach provides results equal to or

superior to those reported for the subvastus or "quadriceps-sparing" techniques; however, it gives the surgeon better visualization while limiting dissection of the quadriceps tendon [24, 25].

The use of smaller, well-designed instruments permits less surgical dissection while avoiding excessive soft tissue retraction. This avoids the need for patellar eversion, thereby reducing the length of the arthrotomy and skin incision. We have found this technique to enhance patient recovery, reduce pain, and improve cosmesis, without compromising the radiographic positioning of the implants or the clinical results.

References

1. Font-Rodriguez DE, Scuderi GR, Insall JN. Survivorship of cemented total knee arthroplasty. Clin Orthop Relat Res 1997;345:79–86
2. Kelly MA, Clarke HD. Long-term results of posterior cruciate substituting total knee arthroplasty. Clin Orthop Relat Res 2002;404:51–57
3. Pavone V, Boettner F, Fickert S, et al. Total condylar knee arthroplasty: a long-term follow-up. Clin Orthop Relat Res 2001;388:18–25
4. Ranawat CS, Flynn WF, Saddler S, et al. Long-term results of the total condylar knee arthroplasty: a 15-year survivorship study. Clin Orthop Relat Res 1993;286:94–102
5. Insall JN. A midline approach to the knee. J Bone Joint Surg 1971;53A:1584–1586
6. Engh GA, Holt BT, Parks NL. A midvastus muscle-splitting approach for total knee arthroplasty. J Arthroplasty 1997;12:322–331
7. Hofmann AA, Plaster RL, Murdock LE. Subvastus (southern) approach for primary total knee arthroplasty. Clin Orthop Relat Res 1991;269:70–77
8. Engh GA, Parks NL. Surgical technique of the midvastus arthrotomy. Clin Orthop Relat Res 1998;351:270–274
9. Dalury DF, Jiranek WA. A comparison of the midvastus and paramedian approaches for total knee arthroplasty. J Arthroplasty 1999;14:33–37
10. White RE, Allman JK, Trauger JA, et al. Clinical comparison of the midvastus and the median parapatellar surgical approaches. Clin Orthop Relat Res 1999;367:117–122
11. Maestro A, Suarez MA, Rodriguez L, et al. The midvastus surgical approach in total knee arthroplasty. Int Orthop Relat Res 2000;24:104–107
12. Bathis H, Perlick L, Blum C, et al. Midvastus approach in total knee arthroplasty: a randomized, double-blinded study on early rehabilitation. Knee Surg Sports Traumatol Arthrosc 2005;13:545–550

13. Parentis MA, Rumi MN, Deol SG, et al. A comparison of the vastus-splitting and median parapatellar approaches in total knee arthroplasty. Clin Orthop Relat Res 1999; 367:101–116

14. Keating EM, Faris PM, Meding JB, et al. Comparison of the midvastus muscle-splitting approach with the median parapatellar approach in total knee arthroplasty. J Arthroplasty 1999;14:29–32

15. Engh GA, Parks NL, Ammeen DJ. Influence of surgical approach on lateral retinacular releases in total knee arthroplasty. Clin Orthop Relat Res 1996;331:56–63

16. Ozkoc G, Hersekli MA, Akpinar S, et al. Time dependent changes in patellar tracking with medial parapatellar and midvastus approaches. Knee Surg Sports Traumatol Arthrosc. 2005;13:654–657

17. Cooper RE Jr, Trinidad G, Buck WR. Midvastus approach in total knee arthroplasty: a description and a cadaveric study determining the distance of the popliteal artery from the patellar margin of the incision. J Arthroplasty 1999;14:505–508

18. Kelly MJ, Rumi MN, Kothari M, et al. Comparison of the vastus-splitting and median parapatellar approaches for primary total knee arthroplasty: a prospective randomized study. J Bone Joint Surg 2006;88A:715–720

19. Macdessi SJ, Manitta MA, Wu A, Reichler B, Haas SB. Electromyographic analysis of the extensor mechanism following a mini-midvastus approach without patellar eversion. Unpublished data

20. Haas SB, Cook S, Beksac B. Minimally invasive total knee replacement through a mini midvastus approach: a comparative study. Clin Orthop Relat Res 2004;428:68–73

21. Haas SB, et al. Follow-up study of minimally invasive total knee replacement through a mini midvastus approach. Unpublished data

22. Laskin RS, Beksac B, Phongjunakorn A, et al. Minimally invasive total knee replacement through a mini-midvastus incision. Clin Orthop Relat Res 2004;428:74–81

23. Laskin RS. Minimally invasive total knee arthroplasty. The results justify its use. Clin Orthop Relat Res 2005;440:54–59

24. Tria AJ Jr, Coon TM. Minimally incision total knee arthroplasty: early experience. Clin Orthop Relat Res 2003;416:185–190

25. Boerger, TO, Aglietti, P, Mondanelli, N, Sensi, L. Mini-subvastus versus medial parapatellar approach in total knee arthroplasty. Clin Orthop Relat Res 2005;440:82–87

Minimally Invasive Total Knee Arthroplasty Suspended Leg Approach and Arthroscopic-Assisted Techniques

9

Peter Bonutti

Minimally invasive total knee arthroplasty (MIS TKA) was developed primarily due to patient demand for less pain, faster recovery, and, it was hoped, improved functional results. Traditional total knee arthroplasty (TKA) consisted of a technique of a supine patient, tourniquet, incision of 6–12 in., median parapatellar approach, everted patella, and dislocated tibiofemoral joint with large bulky instruments that may increase trauma to the soft tissue and prolong recovery.

We began developing MIS knee arthroplasty techniques in 1991 with the goal of reducing overall soft tissue trauma and sparing quadriceps mechanism. After instrumentation and techniques were developed, in 1999 we began performing MIS TKA on selected patients. Our goals were to (1) reduce incision size (12 cm or less); (2) avoid everting the patella; (3) use muscle-sparing techniques – vastus medialis oblique (VMO) snip (mini-midvastus); (4) use downsized instrumentation; and (5) make in situ bone cuts.

In 2001, we first presented our data and evolved into other muscle-sparing techniques [1]. In 2002, we developed the *suspended leg approach*, similar to arthroscopic surgery with the patient's leg hanging distracted by gravity, over the edge of the operating table. The goal was to develop a versatile approach allowing the

surgeon to go from an arthroscopic procedure to a unicompartmental to TKA [2].

In 2003, we began using MIS techniques with computer navigation. We then develop a direct lateral approach with Dr. Michael Mont [3–5]. In 2004, a mini-subvastus approach was developed for exposures [6]. We then used arthroscopic-assisted techniques for visualization of the joint, ligament balancing, and patellar tracking with quadriceps-sparing exposures [7, 8]. In 2005, we utilized these techniques for revision TKA [9]. To date, we have performed nearly 2,000 MIS TKA procedures and are able to do this universally on all patients regardless of age, weight, or deformity.

There is no question that the MIS TKA technique is more difficult and results are only short term. To date, only one article reports a minimum of 2–4 year follow-up with a 97% success rate [3]. We have evaluated the pitfalls and complications of MIS TKA techniques [10] and found that although there is a significant learning curve, the complications once the technique is developed are no different than traditional TKA. This was confirmed in a prospective randomized multicenter clinical trial [11].

Currently, MIS TKA has been classified primarily on the quadriceps exposure: (1) VMO snip (mini-midvastus); (2) "quadriceps saving" (modification of median parapatellar); (3) mini-subvastus; and (4) direct lateral. In all these approaches, the patient is supine, usually with an adjustable leg holder. The incisions are usually shorter than 12 cm, the patella is not everted, and downsized instruments are utilized to make the bone cuts.

P. Bonutti (✉)
Bonutti Clinic, Effingham, IL, USA
e-mail: p@bonutti.net

Department of Orthopaedics, University of Arkansas, Little Rock, AR, USA

G.R. Scuderi and A.J. Tria (eds.), *Minimally Invasive Surgery in Orthopedics: Knee Handbook*, DOI 10.1007/978-1-4614-0679-2_9, © Springer Science+Business Media, LLC 2012

A novel approach, however, utilizing the leg in an arthroscopic position with the leg suspended – hanging over the edge of the table – with various MIS quadriceps exposures has been described [2]. This suspended leg technique has a number of advantages; (1) allowing gravity to distract the soft tissue; (2) enhancing exposure to the posterior joint; (3) allowing the surgeon to be in variable positions (sitting/standing); (4) controlling flexion/extension of the joint; and (5) optimizing patella tracking and soft tissue and ligament balancing both before and after capsular closure (arthroscopic assisted).

This novel approach does have a series of problems. It presents a new view for the reconstructive surgeon; therefore, issues such as patient position, retractor placement, and landmark assessment can be a challenge. Femoral position can be altered by rotating the leg in an adjustable leg support and evaluation of knee extension requires the surgeon to move from a sitting to a standing position. In addition, tibial implantation and cement pressurization require support of the lower extremity during implantation. However, despite these difficulties, the suspended leg approach has been used with quadriceps exposures, computer navigation, and arthroscopic assistance.

Historically, TKA has been performed with the patient supine and the leg in variable positions of flexion and extension [7]. As one progressively flexes and extends the joint, the posterior joint is compressed, which can limit soft tissue visualization, posterior capsular exposure, and, more importantly, accurate ligament and soft tissue balancing.

Arthroscopic knee surgery traditionally is performed with the patient's leg in a leg holder and the joint distracted by gravity. This may enhance joint exposure, visualization, and soft tissue assessment. The surgeon is able to manipulate the extremity from flexion to extension with gravity for an accurate assessment of tissue and ligament balancing. This technique has been utilized in the UKA [12]. Our goal was to assess this suspended approach for TKA and arthroscopic-assisted arthroplasty. This versatile approach may allow different procedures going from arthroscopic to unicompartmental to TKA approach and allowing arthroscopic assistance for this continuum of surgical procedures.

Surgical Technique

The suspended leg approach was originally utilized for TKA in 2002 and was adopted from arthroscopic techniques and approaches. The leg is suspended in a leg holder or padded support (Fig. 9.1). The hip is generally flexed 10–20° and the knee is distracted by gravity and flexed to approximately 90°. This allows body weight and gravity to distract the joint and assess the true deformity, both soft tissue and bone. The soft tissue is stretched by gravity and the skin incision–mobile window can be controlled by variable flexion and extension.

Sterile technique for arthroplasty is critical. We utilize the technique where the patient's leg is sterilely draped directly to the surgeon and to the instrumentation table. The surgeon can be seated or standing and controlling flexion and extension of the joint, optimizing the surgical positioning of the patient's extremity (Fig. 9.2).

The suspended leg technique has been utilized with all of the described MIS muscle-sparing approaches. In all cases, the goal was the overall

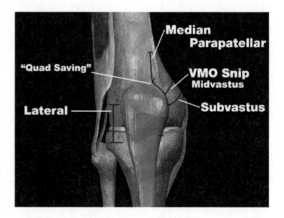

Fig. 9.1 Various quadriceps exposure from the median patellar, quadriceps saving, mini midvastus, mini subvastus, and direct lateral

reduction of soft tissue trauma, avoiding everting the patella, use of downsized instrumentation, and in situ bone cuts (Figs. 9.3 and 9.4).

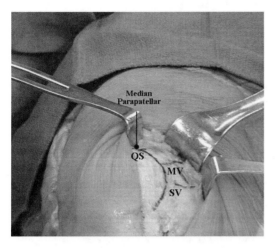

Fig. 9.2 Surgical picture showing the median parapatellar, quadriceps saving (QS), modification of median parapatellar, mini midvastus (MV), and mini subvastus (SV)

A well-trained assistant working with the surgeon is critical. Symbiotic utilization of retractors for exposure, progressively medially then laterally, and allowing a mobile window going from flexion and extension to enhance exposure are necessary.

Downsized "soft tissue-friendly" instrumentation is critical. We use both anterior referencing instrumentation (Fig. 9.5) and posterior referencing (Fig. 9.6). Reducing the bulk of instrumentation allows one to decrease the overall soft tissue envelope required for exposure. This, coupled with the *mobile window*, allows improved visualization and can be further enhanced with arthroscopic assistance.

The suspended leg technique allows gravity to distract the joint, which can be further enhanced by manual distraction or stress medially to laterally to selectively enhance exposure to different segments of the joint (Fig. 9.7). This also enhances soft tissue balancing of the joint. Rather than the surgeon stressing the tibia against

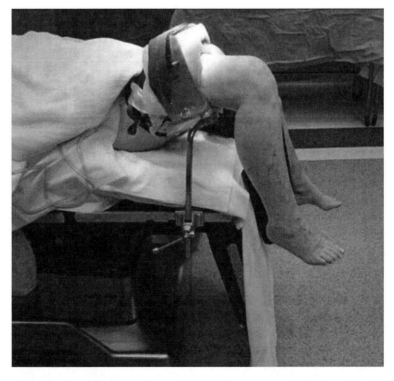

Fig. 9.3 Suspended leg technique. Uses an arthroscopic leg holder versus a padded bolster. The hip is flexed slightly and the knee is suspended with gravity

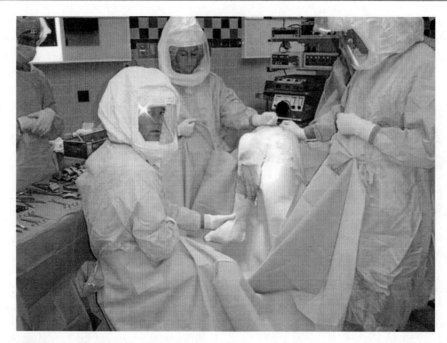

Fig. 9.4 Sterile surgical draping where the patient's leg is suspended and sterile surgical drapes are connected from the patient to the surgeon to the instrumentation table. This allows the surgeon to go from a seated to standing position and mobilize the lower extremity

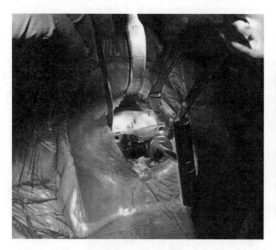

Fig. 9.5 The patella is retracted laterally and the quadriceps mechanism is elevated anteriorly to expose the distal femur

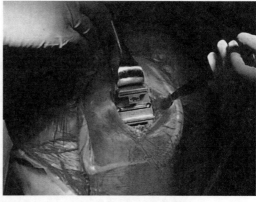

Fig. 9.6 Downsized 4-in-1 cutting instruments

the femur to assess tissue balancing, the patient's leg is flexed and distracted by gravity and can be gently rocked by one or two fingers medially and laterally to assess true ligament balancing (i.e., Rocker Test) (Figs. 9.8 and 9.9). This is physiologic, similar to a patient hanging their leg over the edge of a chair or bed to see if their knee clicks or makes noise in side-to-side motion.

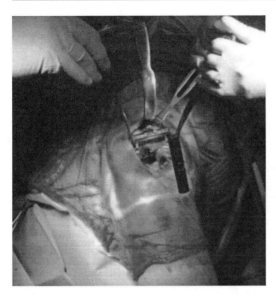

Fig. 9.7 Anterior referencing system

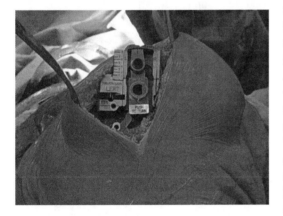

Fig. 9.8 MIS TKA with posterior referencing system

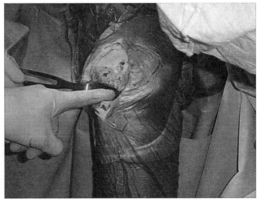

Fig. 9.9 Suspended leg with exposure to the posterior joint. Gravity distracts the joint, enhancing exposure to the posterior joint to improve visualization and access

and after capsular closure with arthroscopic assistance (Fig. 9.10).

The suspended leg approach has also allowed us to utilize arthroscopic assistance in all stages of the procedure (Fig. 9.11). Arthroscopy has a number of advantages and can address many of the difficulties of minimally invasive surgery. Arthroscopy delivers a light source, magnifies the view, allows the surgeon to see around angles (30°/70° arthroscopes), and allows visualization of the joint both before and after capsular closure. The suspended leg technique and arthroscopic assistance can be naturally linked, evolving from diagnostic surgery; ligament reconstruction; biological resurfacing; and arthroscopic-assisted arthroplasty. However, this approach requires further evaluation and new arthroscopic instrumentation (Figs. 9.12 and 9.13).

Appropriate ligament balancing by rocking the leg side to side and rotating with the suspended leg approach is a more a natural and physiologic test and can enhance true ligament balancing.

The patellofemoral joint can also be assessed in a similar fashion going from flexion to extension. We recommend deflating the tourniquet and, with the leg hanging, visualizing the patellofemoral joint. This can be done both before

Results

We performed a retrospective direct patient match study to assess: (1) standard TKA; (2) MIS TKA with a supine approach; and (3) MIS TKA with a suspended leg approach. This is a direct patient-matched study with a standard hospitalization and rehabilitation program. Sixteen patients

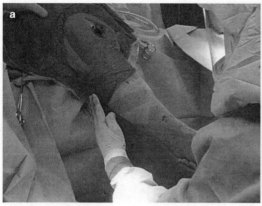 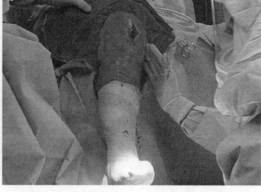

Fig. 9.10 Rocker test. The leg suspended and rocked gently medially and laterally to assess collateral ligament balancing once the trials are in position. One uses a single finger to slide the leg gently medially and laterally to assess ligament balancing with the leg suspended

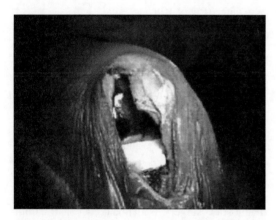

Fig. 9.11 Examination of patellofemoral tracking after implants are in position

(20 TKA) were in each group. The same surgeon, implant (Scorpio TKA, Stryker, Kalamazoo, MI), and rehabilitation protocol were utilized. There was a minimum 3-year follow-up. In group I, the standard technique utilized the 12- to 22-cm incision with an everted patella and median parapatellar approach with traditional instrumentation. In group II, the minimally invasive approach uses the patient supine in an adjustable leg holder with an incision of 6–11 cm, the patella was not everted, and the quadriceps-sparing

technique – VMO snip (mini-midvastus) – was used. In group III, the MIS techniques were used with the suspended leg approach.

Clinical Data

Complications and radiographic analysis were similar in all three groups (Table 9.1). The patients who had MIS techniques, both suspended and supine, had faster recoveries and less postoperative pain. However, in the MIS suspended leg technique, there was a subtle improvement in ligament balancing and patellofemoral tracking observed by the surgeon. Although the sample size was small, there was a slight subjective patient preference for the MIS suspended leg approach [13].

Arthroscopic-Assisted Approach

In an additional study, 22 patients underwent the arthroscopic-assisted suspended leg approach [14]. In these patients, the arthroscopy was

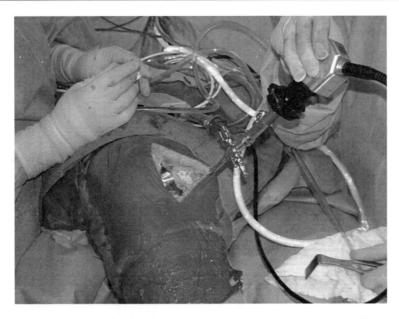

Fig. 9.12 Arthroscopic instruments utilized to examine the joint. Can be used "dry" (without fluid) with the capsule open or with fluid with the capsule closed

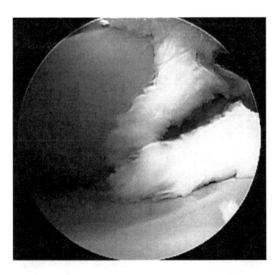

Fig. 9.13 Capsule closed and soft tissue impinging the lateral gutter. This is easily removed

utilized to enhance visualization of the joint for soft tissue and bone removal, implant position, ligament balancing, and patellofemoral tracking both before and after capsular closure. In all patients, arthroscopy was useful to either remove impinging soft tissue, cement, bone fragments, or subtle ligament balancing and/or patellofemoral tracking issues after capsular closure (Fig. 9.14).

Combining the arthroscopic assistance with the suspended leg approach may overall enhance visualization and optimize many of the difficulties associated with MIS TKA techniques – reduced exposure and reduced visualization (Figs. 9.15–9.19).

Conclusion

Although MIS technology is still in its early stages, we recommend an evolutionary approach to all minimally invasive techniques [15]. The surgeon should *evolve*, only change one variable at a time, first learning the downsized instrumentation, then gradually decreasing incision length, then developing muscle-sparing techniques, and then adopting in situ bone cuts.

Table 9.1 Clinical data for study comparing standard TKA, MIS TKA with a supine approach, and MIS TKA with a suspended leg approach

	Group I Standard	Group II MIS	Group III Suspended leg
Clinical data			
Age (years)	75 (65–85)	72 (61–84)	71 (60–83)
Tourniquet time (min)	49 (3961)	54 (5062)	61 (5667)
Knee Society Scores (KSS)			
Range of motion (ROM)			
Preoperative KSS	113 (92–122)	116 (92–125)	118 (86–128)
Postoperative KSS	42 (3254)	41 (3550)	42 (3448)
	96 (80–100)	98 (88–100)	98 (82–100)
Radiographic analysis			
Femoral/tibial valgus	5.6° (2–10°)	5.2° (1–9°)	5.3° (2–9°)
Progressive lucent lines	0	0	0
Postoperative rehabilitation			
Cane 2 weeks	65%	16%	25%
Independent activity	8 weeks (4–16 weeks)	3 weeks (1–7 weeks)	3.5 weeks (2–7 weeks)
Complications			
Lateral release	2 patients	2 patients	1 patient
Manipulations	1 patient	1 patient	1 patient
Re-operation	1 patient—ROM (loss of extension)	0 patients	0 patients

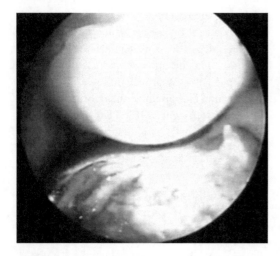

Fig. 9.14 Patellofemoral tracking after capsular closure, arthroscopically visualized

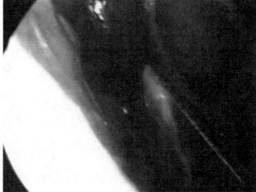

Fig. 9.15 Arthroscopic view of retained posterior cement using 70° scope – later removed

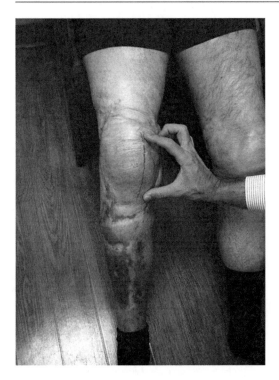

Fig. 9.16 Complex TKA case treated with suspended leg and arthroscopic assistance. The patient had substantial burns to the lower extremity and massive scarring. Suspended leg with MIS TKA approaches and arthroscopic assistance was utilized

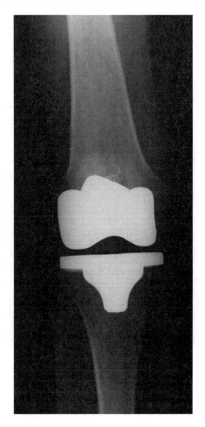

Fig. 9.17 Anteroposterior (AP) view of KM postoperatively

Later, more complex techniques such as suspended leg approaches and arthroscopic assistance may by utilized. Computer navigation may enhance certain issues of alignment and implant position; it does not improve joint visualization, tissue and bone removal, and directly measured patellofemoral tracking ligament balancing. The combination of suspended leg technique, arthroscopic assistance, and computer navigation may optimize all aspects of MIS knee arthroplasty with a goal of improving results [16]. These, combined with future technologies including robotics/haptics for precision bone cuts, modular implants that require optimal implant position, and improved techniques, may afford high-demand patients a return to all functional activities. The goal is not only to improve overall implant survivorship, but to optimize patient satisfaction and functional activity, and even in the highest-demand patients, to give patients optimal surgical results. The suspended leg approach and arthroscopic assistance are two techniques that may enhance results for MIS TKA.

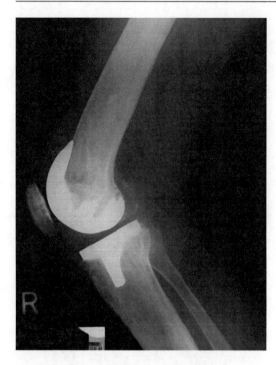

Fig. 9.18 Lateral view of KM postoperatively

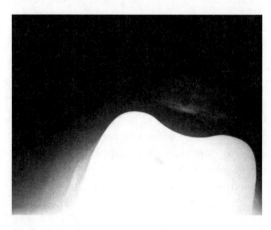

Fig. 9.19 Patellofemoral view of KM postoperatively

References

1. Bonutti P. Minimally Invasive TKR. First Series MIS TKA. Scientific Presentation. LaQuinta, CA, October 2001
2. Bonutti P, Neal D, Kester M. Minimal incision total knee arthroplasty using the suspended leg technique. Orthopedics 2003;26:899–903
3. Bonutti P, Mont M, McMahon M, et al. Minimally invasive total knee arthroplasty. J Bone Joint Surg Am 2004;86:26–32
4. Mont M, Stuchin S, Bonutti P, et al. Different surgical options for monocompartmental OA of the knee: HTO vs. UKA vs. TKA: indications, techniques, results, and controversies. Instr Course Lect 2004;53:265–283
5. Bezwada H, Mont M, Bonutti P, Chauhan S, et al. Minimally invasive lateral approach to total knee arthroplasty. In: Scuderi G, Tria A, Berger R (Eds.), *MIS Techniques in Orthopaedic Surgery*. Springer, New York, Chapter 21:339–348, 2006
6. Bonutti P. Surgical Techniques in Orthopedics. MIS TKA Mini-Subvastus Approach. Standing Room Only AAOS DVD 2005
7. Bonutti P. In: Hozack W, Krismer M, Nogler M, Bonutti P, Rachbauer F, Schaffer J, Donnelly W (Eds.), *Minimally Invasive Total Joint Arthroplasty*. Springer, New York, Chapters:9.1:130–145; 28:284–288; 29: 289–294, 2004
8. Bonutti PM. Minimally invasive total knee arthroplasty. OKU Hip and Knee Reconstruction 3, 8:81–91:01/2006
9. Bonutti P, Seyler TM, Kesler M, et al. Minimally invasive revision total knee arthroplasty. Clin Orthop Relat Res 2006;4469:69–75
10. Bonutti P. Minimally invasive total knee arthroplasty: pitfalls & complications. AAOS Presentation, 2006
11. Kolisek F, Mont M, Bonutti P. MIS TKA prospective randomized multicenter study. JOA, 2006
12. Epinette JA. Personal communication, 1997
13. Bonutti P. The use of the suspended leg minimally invasive technique for total knee arthroplasty. AAOS Presentation, 2005
14. Bonutti P. Arthroscopic assisted total knee arthroplasty. Poster Exhibit. AAOS, 2006
15. Bonutti P, Mont M, Kester M. Minimally invasive total knee arthroplasty: a 10 feature evolutionary approach. Orthop Clin North Am 2004;35:217–226
16. Bonutti P, Mont M. The future of high performance arthroplasty. Semin Arthroplasty, August 2006

Rodney K. Alan and Alfred J. Tria Jr.

Much of the pioneering work for total knee arthroplasty (TKA) took place during the 1970s. For several years, the prosthesis and bearing surfaces were the major focus of efforts to improve the surgery. The result of this evolution is seen in the current success rate of modern TKA [1–4].

During the same period in history, minimally invasive techniques in general surgery and other subspecialties of surgery were beginning to develop. This trend eventually influenced orthopedic surgeons to attempt minimally invasive arthroplasty. The logical first step for minimally invasive TKA was to begin with unicompartmental arthroplasty (UKA). The UKA implant was much smaller than the TKA implant. Repicci pioneered the concept of minimally invasive knee arthroplasty during the early 1990s. He demonstrated that UKA done through a small incision resulted in less blood loss, decreased morbidity, shorter hospitalization, and more rapid recovery [5]. Since his report, other authors have written articles to support the outcome of minimally invasive UKA. Argenson and Price reported decreased morbidity and accelerated rehabilitation

with MIS UKA [6, 7]. After the successful reports of MIS surgery in UKA, investigators began to search for ways to carry out minimally invasive TKA.

The first minimally invasive TKAs were attempted arthroscopically. Caspari, Whipple, and Goble made several attempts to complete the operative procedure with arthroscopic assistance but were unable to perfect the technique and never published any results. When the success of MIS UKA was reported, renewed interest in MIS TKA developed. Implants were modified, instrumentation was made smaller, and new techniques were established.

The development of the quadriceps-sparing TKA began in 2001. The first surgeries were completed in February of 2002 and an early report of the combined results was presented at the Knee Society annual meeting [8]. The paper showed that the arthroplasty was technically possible and reported some early complications. The complications included one transient peroneal nerve palsy, one hematoma, and one knee with decreased range of motion despite a manipulation under anesthesia.

The surgical approach for quadriceps-sparing TKA was not unique at the time it was developed. Many open meniscectomies were performed using the same arthrotomy, but the technique was new for TKA. The designers of the technique did not give the procedure a descriptive name; however, during the first year, the operative procedure began to be called the "quadriceps-sparing" technique. The name is not completely anatomically

R.K. Alan
Department of Surgery, Saint Peter's University Hospital, New Brunswick, NJ, USA

A.J. Tria Jr. (✉)
Institute for Advanced Orthopaedic Study,
The Orthopaedic Center of New Jersey, Somerset, NJ, USA

Department of Orthopedic Surgery, Robert Wood Johnson Medical School, Piscataway, NJ, USA
e-mail: atriajrmd@aol.com

correct. The medial arthrotomy extends from the superior pole of the patella to 2 cm below the tibiofemoral joint line. The vastus medialis inserts along the medial side of the patella, and, in some cases, the muscle insertion is as low as the midpoint of the patella. Thus, the arthrotomy does divide the insertion in some cases; and, therefore, the technique is not always quadriceps sparing. With this proviso, the authors have continued to call the procedure "quadriceps sparing" because the name and the technique have become synonymous.

Other minimally invasive approaches have been described for TKA. Tenholder et al. used a minimally invasive medial parapatellar approach and reported that patients with this approach required fewer transfusions and achieved better flexion [9]. The subvastus approach avoids disruption of the quadriceps mechanism and may provide more rapid recover after TKA [10–13]. Boerger et al. reported less blood loss, less pain, greater motion, faster straight leg raising, but more complications with a minimally invasive subvastus TKA [14].

A vastus-splitting approach has been described and used successfully in more than 420 minimally invasive TKAs by Bonutti et al. [15] Laskin reported that patients with an MIS midvastus approach required less analgesic drugs in the perioperative period, regained flexion faster, and achieved functional milestones more rapidly when compared with a matched group of patients with standard TKA [16]. Because there are different types of minimally invasive TKA techniques, it is difficult to compare one MIS procedure to another. The quadriceps-sparing procedure is the least invasive of the techniques. It is more difficult to perform and requires more of the surgeon and the patient.

Defining Minimally Invasive

Minimally invasive surgery of the knee represents a spectrum of approaches and exposures. All of the skin incision lengths are shorter than the standard incision but the skin incision itself does not identify the MIS procedure. The ideal minimally invasive knee replacement should limit the skin incision, limit the disruption of the quadriceps mechanism, and avoid eversion of the patella while maintaining the quality and safety of standard TKA. In retrospect, it now appears that eversion of the patella is a central factor that may very well be the common defining point for the MIS procedures [17].

Preoperative Evaluation

Patients must have radiographically confirmed symptomatic arthritis that has not responded to conservative measures. Age considerations do not differ for the quadriceps-sparing technique. Initially, the procedure was twice as long as the standard operation and the senior author deferred using the technique in patients older than the age of 80 years because of the increased anesthetic exposure. Now that the operative time is almost the same as the standard approach, this limitation has been somewhat relaxed.

The patient should be capable of performing the physical therapy regimen after the surgery and should understand the general goals of the MIS operation. The knee should have no significant previous arthrotomy or periarticular scarring because this makes the approach much more difficult. The clinical deformity should not exceed 15° in any given plane and the knee should have a minimum of 105° of motion. Obesity does play a role in the selection process but refers only to the local anatomy of the knee. If the circumference of the lower leg at the level of the knee is much smaller than the length of the thigh, the procedure will be much easier. The authors are trying to develop a meaningful ratio of these two measurements and it does appear that a three to one ratio (thigh length versus knee circumference) is ideal.

There are some factors that increase the difficulty of the surgical procedure but are not absolute contraindications. The rheumatoid knee is not ideal because the bone tends to be osteoporotic and may be injured at the time of the prosthetic insertion. Patella baja makes it difficult to retract the patella across the lateral femoral condyle. The vastus medialis may be very well developed in some muscular males and the insertion can be as low as the mid portion of the patella. When this occurs, it is difficult to retract the medial capsule. The largest femoral components from any design line will often require an extension of the capsular incision just to accommodate the prosthetic size.

The quadriceps-sparing technique is not meant for all knees. Strict criteria should certainly be observed at the initiation of the surgical approach so that the result will be rewarding both for the surgeon and the patient. The authors typically use the approach for 25–30% of all TKAs in a given year.

Surgical Technique

The patient is placed supine and an arterial tourniquet is applied to the upper thigh. A leg holder is used for the quadriceps-sparing technique because the bone cuts are made in varying positions of flexion and extension and the holder expedites the positioning (Fig. 10.1). A curvilinear skin incision is made from the superior pole of the patella to the tibial joint line just medial to the patella and patella tendon (Fig. 10.2). The arthrotomy is made in line with the skin incision

beginning at the superomedial border of the patella, where the vastus medialis typically inserts, and ending 2 cm below the tibial joint line. Both the varus and valgus knee can be replaced through the medial arthrotomy; however, a lateral arthrotomy can also be used with elevation of the iliotibial band from Gerdy's tubercle posteriorly. The arthrotomy is not extended proximally into the quadriceps tendon, the vastus medialis, or the subvastus interval.

The extremity is brought into full extension and the patellar fat pad is excised. The patellar thickness is recorded and the MIS patellar guide is used to remove a measured amount of bone (Fig. 10.3). Alternately, the patella surface can be resected using a freehand technique; but the position of the patella is not typical and somewhat awkward. A metal protector is placed over the patellar surface for the remainder of the procedure (Fig. 10.4). Early patellar resection is not mandatory, but it increases the overall working room within the knee joint, thus making it easier for later steps in the procedure.

With the knee remaining in full extension, the anterior surface of the femur is cleared to permit subsequent sizing and positioning of the anterior femoral cut. The knee is flexed to 45°, and the

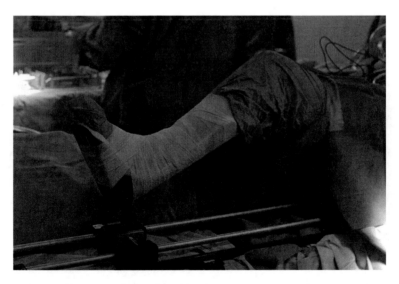

Fig. 10.1 The leg holder (Innovative Medical Products, Plainville, CT, USA) facilitates positioning of the knee throughout the range of motion

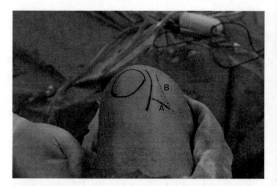

Fig. 10.2 The MIS incision. "*A*" is the tibiofemoral joint line and "*B*" is the outline of the medial femoral condyle

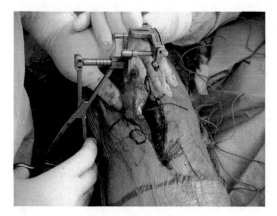

Fig. 10.3 The patellar clamp leaves a predetermined thickness for resurfacing (Zimmer Orthopedics, Warsaw, IN, USA)

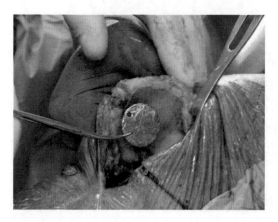

Fig. 10.4 The metal protector is centered on the cut surface of the patella

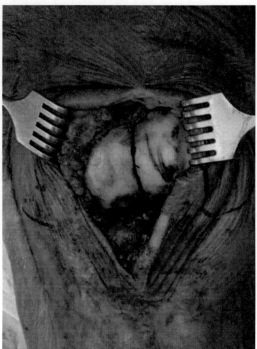

Fig. 10.5 Whiteside's line is drawn for rotational referencing for the femoral cuts

anterior and posterior cruciate ligaments are resected from the intercondylar notch. The author's preference is a posterior cruciate-substituting knee replacement for both minimally invasive TKA and standard TKA. However, cruciate-substituting and cruciate-retaining knee replacements are both amenable to the quadriceps-sparing approach [18].

The anteroposterior (AP) axis line of Whiteside's is drawn (Fig. 10.5) and an intramedullary rod is introduced into the femur through a hole just above the intercondylar notch. A modified intramedullary cutting guide is used to make the distal femoral cut in a medial to lateral direction. In order to complete the distal femoral cut, the intramedullary reference must be removed. The cutting guide remains secured to the medial aspect of the distal femur, and the resection is continued until the saw abuts the cutting guide. In patients with a small femur, the entire resection can be completed. In patients with large femurs, the cutting guide is removed, and the resection is completed by freehand technique, taking care not to violate the lateral capsule.

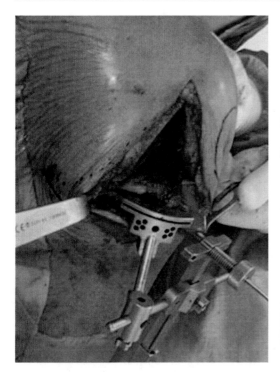

Fig. 10.6 The extramedullary tibial cutting guide is medially based

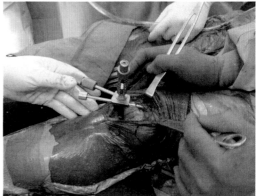

Fig. 10.7 The femoral cutting guide references the posterior femoral condyles and locates the site for the anterior cut

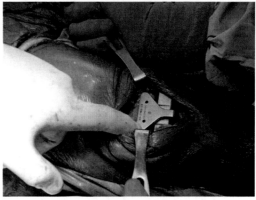

Fig. 10.8 The femoral finishing block is centered medial to lateral and pinned into position

The proximal tibial cut is completed using a standard extramedullary cutting guide with the cutting attachment biased toward the medial side of the tibia (Fig. 10.6). The proximal tibial bone can usually be removed in a single piece. A spacer block can be inserted into the extension gap and the overall alignment and balance of the knee can be evaluated. Ligamentous releases can be completed at this juncture without difficulty because the bone resections leave approximately 20 mm of space in full extension.

The anterior aspect of the distal femur is cut using a guide that references the posterior femoral condyles and the anteroposterior axis (Fig. 10.7). A shelf is attached to the appropriate femoral finishing block and the shelf is set on the anterior femoral surface in full extension. The finishing block is centered on the distal femur and pinned in place (Fig. 10.8). The knee is flexed to 70° and the femoral finishing cuts and peg holes are completed. The flexion gap can now be compared with the extension gap and adjustments can be made in the standard fashion.

The proximal tibia finishing guide has two deployable posterior pins that reference the cortex of the tibia (Fig. 10.9). The tray is centered medial to lateral and rotated to reference the tibial tubercle, the femoral box cut, and the malleoli of the ankle. The broaching is completed in the standard fashion.

If the patella is resurfaced, the metal protector is removed and the pegs holes are completed.

The tibial tray, femoral component, polyethylene insert, and trial patella are inserted in order. Patellar tracking, ligament balance, range of motion, and overall knee alignment are confirmed and the surfaces are prepared for cementing. Palacos cement is preferred because of its prolonged "doughy" state. There are MIS tibial

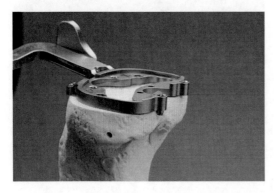

Fig. 10.9 Tibial cutting guide has deployable pins that can be used to hook the posterior cortex of the femur

components now available with shortened intramedullary stems to facilitate insertion of the component (Fig. 10.10). While these are helpful, they are not absolutely necessary.

After cementing is completed and excess cement removed, the polyethylene insert is locked into position. The tourniquet is released and hemostasis is achieved by electrocautery. Surgical drains can be used if desired and closure is completed in the standard fashion.

Perioperative Management

The authors' postoperative management has evolved during the past 5 years. The original protocol shortened the hospital stay without making any other changes [8]. Minor changes have been

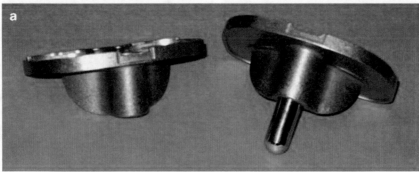

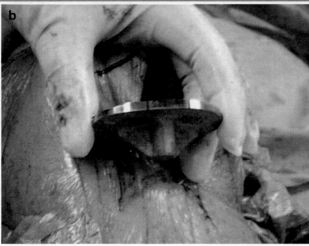

Fig. 10.10 (**a**) This MIS modular tibial component can be inserted with or without the pin (MIS tibia, Zimmer Orthopedics, Warsaw, IN, USA). (**b**) This MIS tibia is a single component with a shortened intramedullary stem (MIS tibia, Smith and Nephew, Memphis, TN, USA)

made in the pain management but peripheral blocks have not been incorporated in our center because of the concern for muscle paralysis. The patients no longer donate autologous blood and they can go home as soon as the first day after surgery. Full weight-bearing ambulation and range of motion exercises are routinely initiated within hours after the operation. Low molecular weight heparin (LMWH) is used for deep vein thrombosis (DVT) prophylaxis, and all patients undergo a Doppler study of both lower extremities before stopping the LMWH at 12–14 days after surgery.

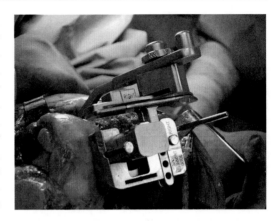

Fig. 10.11 The standard intramedullary guide has been downsized and the anterior cutting slot modified to fit into the smaller incision

Technical Pearls

Patient selection is important for the success of the procedure. The thinner patient, with a good range of motion, and some laxity of the joint is an ideal candidate.

Positioning the knee in varying degrees of flexion throughout the procedure is an important point that differentiates minimally invasive TKA from the standard TKA that is typically performed in full extension or 90° of flexion. The leg holder allows changing the position of the knee throughout the operation and does not require another assistant.

Initially, the quadriceps-sparing TKA required special instrumentation. The authors recognized the hesitation of surgeons to adopt radically different instruments and have now developed instruments that are modifications of standard existing designs (Fig. 10.11). The distal femoral cut can now be made from anterior to posterior. The femoral finishing block is a standard shape with an anterior shelf (Fig. 10.12). The tibial guide cuts more from anterior to posterior and the tibial trays can now be positioned on the cut surface without using posterior hooks.

There are some minimally invasive tibial components available that have an abbreviated intramedullary stem. The shorter stem does facilitate insertion of the component; however, as the authors have increased their experience with the MIS exposures, the need for the modified components decreases. The high-flex femoral component

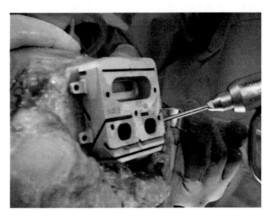

Fig. 10.12 A standard cutting block can be used with the edges cut down to fit into the smaller incision

(Legacy High Flex, Zimmer, Warsaw, IN, USA) removes 2 mm of additional bone from the posterior aspect of the femur and this also increases some of the working space in the knee.

Results

The senior author has completed more than 500 quadriceps-sparing TKAs. The incisions have been extended on six occasions; four for implanting large femoral components, one for gaining additional exposure in an obese patient, and one for bleeding from the middle geniculate artery. The operative times have gradually decreased and the procedure is now routinely completely in less than 60 min. The blood loss is less than the standard TKA, the length of stay is less, and the pain is less. There is greater motion in the early postoperative period, but this difference diminishes over time. At a minimum of 2-year follow-up, patients with quadriceps-sparing TKA have more motion, but only by a few degrees. While this does not represent a clinically significant difference at this time, it does give a positive effect for future development.

The radiographic analysis of the results has shown that the quadriceps-sparing technique does have more outliers than the standard approach [19]. An outlier was defined as 4° or more outside the ideal alignment, size difference of 4 mm for a component, or 2 mm of femoral notching. There were 13 outliers in 32 MIS TKAs and 5 outliers in 38 standard TKAs. There was no statistical difference in coronal plane alignment between the two groups and, with 2–4 years of follow-up, there were no repeat surgeries or component failures in either group.

The results of quadriceps-sparing TKA have paralleled other investigators who have reported results of minimally invasive TKAs. Laskin et al. and Haas et al. have reported results of their minimally invasive TKA and found greater range of motion and excellent Knee Society scores at short-term follow-up [16, 20]. With the quadriceps-sparing technique, there were no statistically significant differences in Knee Society scores when compared with standard TKA. The quadriceps-sparing group had slightly better scores, but the difference was neither clinically nor statistically different.

Summary

The impact of minimally invasive TKA continues to generate much discussion and controversy all over the world. Early results of the technique are encouraging, but long-term data is still lacking. Patient interest continues to be high and patients request the procedure because they look for less postoperative pain and earlier return to function.

The quadriceps-sparing TKA addresses the patient's needs and desires. The technique does need to be further refined and the accuracy improved. The authors continued to address these issues. The instruments have been modified so that they are more user friendly; the postoperative management is constantly refined; and computer navigation has been incorporated to address the accuracy.

References

1. National Institutes of Health. NIH Consensus Statement on total knee replacement December 8–10, 2003. J Bone Joint Surg Am. 2004;86-A(6):1328–35
2. Ritter MA, Herbst SA, Keating EM, PM, Meding JB. Long-term survival analysis of a posterior cruciate-retaining total condylar total knee arthroplasty. Clin Orthop Relat Res. 1994 Dec;(309):136–45
3. Scott RD, Volatile TB. Twelve years' experience with posterior cruciate-retaining total knee arthroplasty. Clin Orthop Relat Res. 1986 Apr;(205):100–7
4. Stern S, Insall J. Posterior stabilized prosthesis. Results after follow-up of nine to twelve years. J Bone Joint Surg Am. 1992;74(7):980–6
5. Repicci JA, Eberle RW. Minimally invasive surgical technique for unicondylar knee arthroplasty. J South Orthop Assoc. 1999;8(1):20–7
6. Argenson JN, Flecher X. Minimally invasive unicompartmental knee arthroplasty. Knee. 2004;11(5):341–7
7. Price AJ, Webb J, Topf H, Dodd CA, Goodfellow JW, Murray DW; Oxford Hip and Knee Group. Rapid recovery after oxford unicompartmental arthroplasty through a short incision. J Arthroplasty. 2001;16(8):970–6
8. Tria AJ Jr, Coon TM. Minimal incision total knee arthroplasty: early experience. Clin Orthop Relat Res. 2003 Nov;(416):185–90
9. Tenholder M, Clarke HD, Scuderi GR. Minimal-incision total knee arthroplasty: the early clinical experience. Clin Orthop Relat Res. 2005 Nov;(440):67–76
10. Faure BT, Benjamin JB, Lindsey B, Volz RG, Schutte D. Comparison of the subvastus and paramedian surgical approaches in bilateral knee arthroplasty. J Arthroplasty. 1993;8(5):511–6
11. Hofmann AA, Plaster RL, Murdock LE. Subvastus (Southern) approach for primary total knee arthroplasty. Clin Orthop Relat Res. 1991 Aug;(269):70–7
12. Matsueda M, Gustilo, RB. Subvastus and medial parapatellar approaches in total knee arthroplasty. Clin Orthop Relat Res. 2000 Feb;(371):161–8
13. Roysam GS, Oakley MJ. Subvastus approach for total knee arthroplasty: a prospective, randomized, and observer-blinded trial. J Arthroplasty. 2001;16(4):454–7
14. Boerger TO, Aglietti P, Mondanelli N, Sensi L. Mini-subvastus versus medial parapatellar approach in total knee arthroplasty. Clin Orthop Relat Res. 2005 Nov;(440):82–7

15. Bonutti PM, Mont MA, Kester MA. Minimally invasive total knee arthroplasty: a 10-feature evolutionary approach. Orthop Clin North Am. 2004;35(2):217–26
16. Laskin RS, Beksac B, Phongjunakorn A, Pittors K, Davis J, Shim JC, Pavlov H, Petersen M. Minimally invasive total knee replacement through a mini-midvastus incision: an outcome study. Clin Orthop Relat Res. 2004 Nov;(428):74–81
17. Laskin RS. *Acquired patella baja after total knee replacement may be related to patellar tendon eversion.* Presented at the Annual Closed meeting of the Knee Society, September 29, 2006, Alexandria, VA

18. Berger RA, Sanders S, Gerlinger T, Della Valle C, Jacobs JJ, Rosenberg AG. Outpatient total knee arthroplasty with a minimally invasive technique. J Arthroplasty. 2005;20(7 Suppl 3):33–8
19. Chen AF, Alan RK, Redziniak DE, Tria AJ Jr. Quadriceps sparing total knee replacement. The initial experience with results at two to four years. J Bone Joint Surg Br. 2006;88B(11):1448–53
20. Haas SB, Cook S, Beksac B. Minimally invasive total knee replacement through a mini midvastus approach: a comparative study. Clin Orthop Relat Res. 2004 Nov;(428):68–73

Minimally Invasive Quadriceps-Sparing Total Knee Replacement Preserving the Posterior Cruciate Ligament

11

Richard A. Berger and Aaron G. Rosenberg

Minimally invasive has been used to describe a wide spectrum of knee replacement procedures. This spectrum starts with a small skin incision with a standard incision into the capsular and the quadriceps muscle and includes patellar eversion. The spectrum currently ends with a small skin incision with a minimal capsular incision without quadriceps muscle violation and no patellar eversion. This is currently called the quadriceps-sparing or capsular-only approach.

Whatever the definition used, minimally invasive knee replacement can be done and has been shown to be beneficial to patients by minimizing surgical trauma, pain, and recovery [1–10]. All of the varied minimally invasive techniques share common elements of reducing the trauma necessary for exposure, component alignment, soft tissue balance, and component fixation. Ultimately, these benefits of minimally invasive knee replacement result in a more satisfied patient.

Additionally, to achieve potential rapid recovery that a minimally invasive technique can offer, the entire traditional perioperative pathway needs to be expedited. By combining one of these minimally invasive total knee replacement techniques with new pathways that expedite the entire recovery process, rapid recovery is not only possible, but outpatient total knee replacement is

both possible and is currently being performed at our hospital daily [1–3].

Wherever approach you ultimately choose, minimally invasive knee replacement has to adhere to the basic principles of knee replacement: proper alignment, proper balance, and good fixation. In addition, any new technique should not increase the complication rate compared with traditional knee replacement and must not compromise the outcome or longevity of a traditional knee replacement.

Indications

The limited mobility of the patella and extensor mechanism, the inability to evert the patella, and the inability to anteriorly dislocate the tibia in hyperflexion that result from the small retinacular arthrotomy make this approach the most challenging of all of the minimally invasive total knee approaches. However, with proper experience, the quadriceps-sparing approach can be used in almost all patients undergoing traditional total knee replacement. The approach allows for the exposure, proper resections, proper ligamentous balancing, and component insertion in most patients undergoing primary total knee arthroplasty (TKA).

The initial attempts at the quadriceps-sparing approach should be restricted to the easiest cases; thin female patients with good range of motions and lax tissues. Patients with patella alta and minimal varus-valgus deformity are also easier

R.A. Berger (✉) • A.G. Rosenberg
Department of Orthopaedic Surgery, Rush Medical College,
Rush-Presbyterian-St. Luke's Medical Center,
Chicago, IL, USA
e-mail: r.a.berger@sbcglobal.net

cases for learning the technique. As with all new approach in orthopedics, there is a learning curve to this quadriceps-sparing approach. Alternative positioning and retraction using the mobile window to gain appropriate exposure is key. The more of the procedure that can be done in extension, the easier it is to mobilize the patella and extensor mechanism. Once a surgeon has gained sufficient experience and comfort with the procedure, then the management of cases that are more difficult is possible: heavy male patients with poor range of motion and stiff tissues. In addition, cases with patellar baja and severe varus–valgus deformities are also possible. In our experience, even patients with moderate to severe deformities are candidates for the quadriceps-sparing approach.

The type and size of the component also influence the difficulty of the technique. Due the small arthrotomy and the inability to mobilize the extensor mechanism in flexion, this approach is more difficult in patients with larger femoral components. The inability to sublux the tibia makes it is extremely difficult to use a monoblock tibia or large-stemmed tibial components. This approach is easiest for primary knee arthroplasty using a low-profile tibial component or a modular tibial component.

Lastly, this minimally invasive approach can be increased to gain exposure in a stepwise fashion if difficulties are encountered. A very low threshold for lengthening the arthrotomy should be maintained at all times, especially while learning minimally invasive approaches. The quadriceps-sparing arthrotomy may be easily extended in a step-wise fashion, into a medial parapatellar arthrotomy or into the midvastus or subvastus interval. Therefore, there are easy methods to increase exposure should intraoperative difficulty arise.

Patient Positioning

Unlike traditional approaches where the majority of the procedure is done in flexion, the quadriceps-sparing approach requires more of the procedure to be performed in relative extension. Furthermore, this approach, as with

most minimally invasive approaches, requires constantly flexing and extending the knee to gain the best exposure for each step; small changes in the flexion of the knee result in large changes in exposure. Furthermore, while performing a femoral preparation with the approach, which is normally done in hyperflexion in traditional TKA, the knee should be extended as much as possible without interference with the cutting block. Therefore, a leg holder that will accommodate variations in positioning for incremental changes in knee flexion is very helpful.

As with a traditional TKA, the patient is positioned supine, with a bump under the ischium to tilt the pelvis and allow the knee to stay vertical during the surgery. The extremity is prepared and draped in standard fashion, including the incorporation of a leg holder to allow for incremental positioning of the flexed extremity. A thigh tourniquet is helpful to limit blood loss. Lastly, although this technique for total knee replacement can be done with one assistant, two assistants make the procedure much easier for the surgeon. However, care should be taken to ensure that the two assistants are not applying traction to both sides of the incision at once, which would potentially injure the tissue and inhibit the exposure.

Exposure

Proper positioning of the incision is important for maximal exposure. With the knee at 70° flexion, the medial patellar border, joint line, and tibial tuberosity are usually easy to palpate. A curvilinear incision that begins at the superomedial patella and ends at the medial edge of the tibial tuberosity is drawn (Fig. 11.1). Throughout its course, the incision curves; at its midpoint, it is 1 cm medial patella.

After the incision is made through the skin and subcutaneous tissue, a self-retractor is placed. Two curved joint retractors are placed at the superior and medial edge of the incision, revealing the distal extent of the vastus medialis oblique (VMO), which is seen in the superior medial aspect of the incision. At this point, the entire extent of the joint capsule from the superior pole

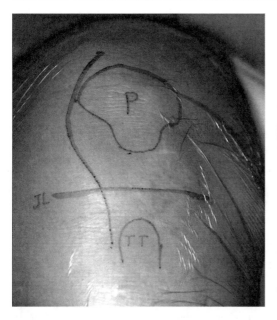

Fig. 11.1 Skin incision for the minimally invasive, quadriceps-sparing, total knee arthroplasty. *P* patella; *JL* joint line; *TT* tibial tubercle

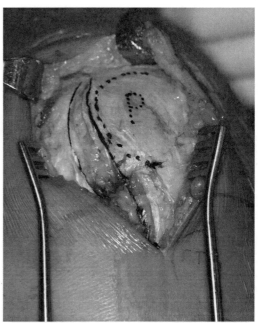

Fig. 11.2 Arthrotomy for the minimally invasive, quadriceps-sparing total knee arthroplasty

of the patella down to the medial edge of the tibial tubercle is exposed.

The borders of the patella, the distal extent of the VMO, and the medial border of the tibial tubercle is identified. The distal VMO insertion varies, with lower insertions on muscular patients and male patients. An arthrotomy is made from the superior pole of the patella, extending along the medial border of the patella, to the medial aspect of the tibial tubercle, avoiding the patellar tendon (Fig. 11.2). The arthrotomy is extended distally to 1 cm inferior to the tibial plateau. Care is taken to leave enough retinaculum between the arthrotomy and VMO to prevent tearing of the arthrotomy into the VMO. The exposure is aided in some patients, especially in muscular males, by back cutting the retinaculum 1–2 cm. This is done distal to the VMO, approximately 1/2 cm distal to the edge of the VMO. This back cut should not extend more than 2 cm. If this back cut is made, the inferior medial retinaculum is tagged with a stitch, which helps as a retractor.

With the arthrotomy completed, blunt dissection is used to define the plane between the medial retinaculum and synovium. Then a portion of the superior medial synovium is excised, thus providing excellent exposure to the medial condyle. A retractor is positioned around the medial condyle, and it retracts the medial collateral ligament (MCL) and medial retinaculum. The anterior insertion of the medial meniscus is then detached. This then exposes the medial femoral condyle. As with a traditional exposure, the deep MCL is released from the proximal medial tibial plateau. This release may be extended with a curved osteotome to achieve the appropriate ligamentous release. Finally, the leg can be extended and externally rotated to extend the medial release posteriorly. In this position, the medial osteophytes on the tibial plateau are removed.

With the knee in extension, using blunt dissection, the space between the fat pad and patellar tendon is developed and a knee joint retractor is placed in the plane. Scissors are used to extend this plane and resect the attachments of the fat pad to the patella and tibia, thus excising a large portion of the fat pad. The knee is then flexed to 70°. A retractor exposes the medial femoral condyle and the medial osteophytes on the femoral

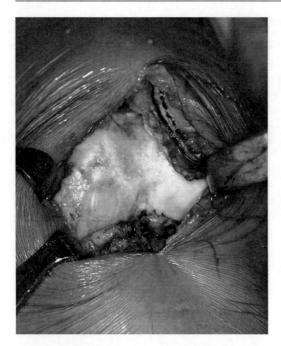

Fig. 11.3 Initial exposure of the knee showing the distal femoral condyle

condyle are removed. Finally, the anterior cruciate ligament (ACL) and meniscal attachments are incised to mobilize the tibia, which also facilitates the tibial cut. With the knee flexed to 70°, a double-pronged Hohmann retractor is placed over the lateral femoral condyle that gently retracts the patella laterally (Fig. 11.3).

Distal Femoral Resection

During a conventional total knee replacement, the distal femoral cut is made from anterior to posterior. This step is traditionally aided by hyperflexion of the knee. However, the quadriceps-sparing approach requires this step to be performed in less flexion, usually approximately 70–80°. In this position, the distal cut must be made from the medial side, cutting from medial to lateral; this avoids the extensor mechanism. More than 70–80° of flexion tightens the extensor mechanism, making this resection more difficult.

A double-pronged Hohmann retractor is placed over the lateral femoral condyle and gently

retracts the patella laterally, exposing the intercondylar notch (Fig. 11.3). In this position, with the intercondylar notch exposed, an 8-mm hole is made with a drill in the axis of the femoral canal (Fig. 11.4).

Through this hole, the distal femoral cutting guide will be inserted into the femoral canal. The cutting guide is chosen to match the difference between the mechanical axis and anatomic axis. In this case, a 5° distal femoral guide is chosen. Prior to inserting, the L-shaped cutting guide is attached to the distal femoral cutting guide. Then the intermedullary rod is inserted into the distal femoral canal and the flat plate is seated against the medial femoral condyle. This will resect 10 mm of bone from the medial condyle plate at the specific valgus angle. The L-shaped cutting slot is seated against the medial and superior edge of the medial femoral condyle. This is done at approximately 70–80° of flexion. This cutting guide is designed to avoid the intact quadriceps tendon, cutting the distal femur from the medial aspect of the knee. The guide must be seated against the medial femoral condyle. Retraction of the medial soft tissue facilitates insertion (Fig. 11.5).

The distal femoral cutting guide is secured against the medial condyle with threaded screw pins. The orthogonal orientations of the screws hold the cutting block securely and prevent angular change during the cutting of the distal femur. The distal condyles are resected using an oscillating saw from medial to lateral; first the medial condyle is resected then the lateral condyle is resected. The medial condyle is resected using the "L" shaped guide from anterior to posterior. The very posterior aspect of the distal lateral condyle can then resected with the intramedullary rod in place. The cut is made as shown in Fig. 11.5. The central and anterior portion of the distal lateral femoral condyle cannot be resected until the intramedullary rod is removed. At this point, the L-shaped cutting block is detached from the intramedullary rod and the rod is removed. With the L-shaped cutting block remaining pinned to the medial femoral condyle, the central aspects of the lateral condyle can then resected (Fig. 11.5). During this step, care is

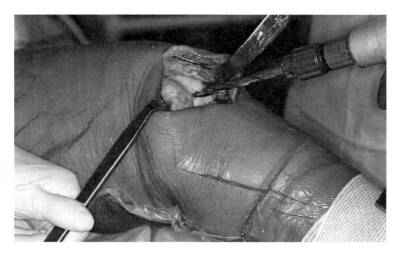

Fig. 11.4 Drill the intramedullary hole for the distal femur. Extending the knee slightly relaxes the extensor mechanism, facilitating the process

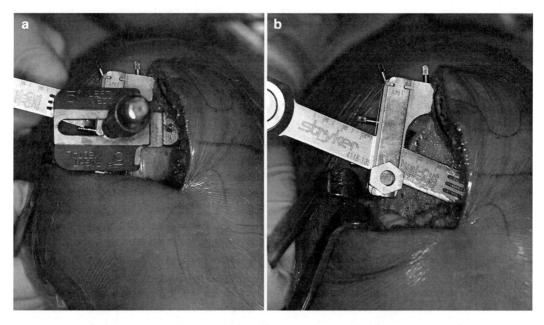

Fig. 11.5 Cutting the distal femur. (**a**) Distal femoral cutting guide in place. After the medial condyle resected, the posterior distal lateral femur is cut obliquely from the anterior medial side. (**b**) L-shaped cutting block as a guide for the central portion of the lateral distal femoral

taken not to cut the lateral retinaculum; this is aided by cutting from anterior to posterior and retractor may be placed over the lateral knee to protect the lateral retinaculum as the lateral femoral condyle is resected. After the L-shaped cutting block is removed the anterior aspect of the distal lateral condyle is resected with the knee in extension with a reciprocating saw. The knee in extension allows better expose the lateral condyle so it can be resected and removed.

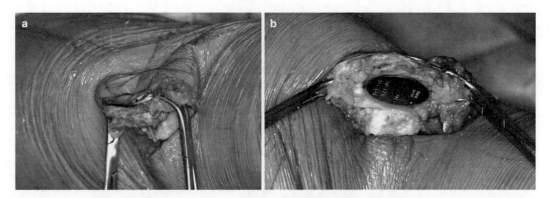

Fig. 11.6 Resecting the patella. (**a**) Distal femur in extension. The patella is seen and resected. (**b**) A patellar protector is placed

Preparing the Patella

The patella cannot be everted. However, after the distal femoral condyles are removed, the knee is placed in slight hyperextension. This hyperextension allows the patellar to be tilted between 45° and 90° from the coronal axis. This is the reason that the patella is resected after the distal femoral condyles. In addition, the unresected patella prevents the patella from unintentional damage during the distal femoral resection.

In this position, one towel clip is placed on the superior pole and one towel clip is placed on the inferior poles of the patella. These two clips allow the patella to be tilted between 45° and 90°. This is adequate exposure for the patellar resection (Fig. 11.6). Patellar eversion is not needed to resect the patella. The patellar thickness is measured with a caliper and the patella is resected to recreate the patellar thickness with the implant in place. The patellar component size is chosen to cover the resected surface of the patella without overhanging. The patellar bone is then prepared with drill holes. Lastly, a patellar protector is placed on the resected surface to prevent damage to the soft cancellous bone of the patella with subsequent retractors (Fig. 11.6).

Preparing the Tibia

The tibia is resected with the knee in relative extension. A small bolster is placed under the proximal tibia, positioning the knee in approximately 15° of flexion (Fig. 11.7). This position takes tension off the extensor mechanism and allows visualization and access to the proximal tibia. This position facilitates placement of the tibial cutting guide beneath the patellar tendon into the proximal tibia. The tibial cutting guide is positioned just proximal to the tibial tubercle, along the medial tibial tubercle. With the overall alignment and slope of the tibial guide set, the guide is set to achieve the correct level of tibial plateau resection. A retractor is placed on the medial plateau to protect the medial collateral ligament and a second retractor is used to retract the patellar tendon laterally (Fig. 11.7). Then, an oscillating saw is used to resect the proximal tibia. While most of the resection in completed under direct visualization, care must be taken resecting the posterolateral tibia where either a retractor or tactile sense can be used to avoid cutting through the posterior-lateral capsule and injuring posterolateral structures.

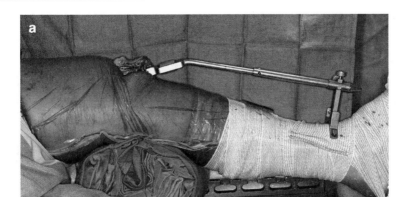

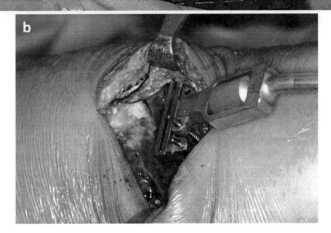

Fig. 11.7 Tibial resection. (**a**) Positioning for the tibial cut with a bolster. (**b**) The extended position relaxes the extensor mechanism and retractors protect the soft tissue

After resection, the medial edge of the tibial resection is grasped with a Kocher. The Kocher is used externally to rotate the fragment as the proximal attachments are sequentially released. With the ACL and meniscal attachments divided, the tibial fragment is easily removed. After the tibial fragment is removed, the leg is placed into full extension. A laminar spreader is then used in the extension space to expose the menisci. In this position, the menisci are easily seen and completely resected (Fig. 11.8). Any additional soft tissue releases to balance the knee can be easily accomplished in this extended position where both the lateral and medial structures are easily seen (Fig. 11.8). Lastly, a spacer block is used in extension to gauge the extension gap and to assess the soft tissue balancing.

Completing the Femur

Completion of the femur requires the knee to be positioned in 80–90° of flexion. A double-pronged Hohmann retractor is placed over the medial femoral condyle and another is placed over the lateral femoral condyle; this exposes the femur. The final femoral sizing guide is then positioned on the distal femur with the two skids placed under the posterior condyles (Fig. 11.9). This sets rotation at 3° external to the posterior condyles. This position usually coincides with Whitesides' line in varus knees; however, in valgus knees, the posterior condyles will internally rotate the guide. Therefore, in valgus knees, the guide must be externally rotated from the femoral condyles to align with Whitesides' line. After the guide is

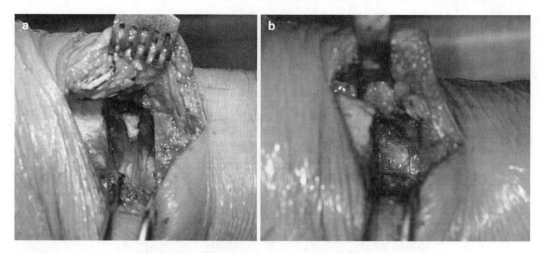

Fig. 11.8 (**a**) The lateral menisci is seen well in full extension. (**b**) After the menisci are removed, the lateral structures are easily visualized and can be subsequently released

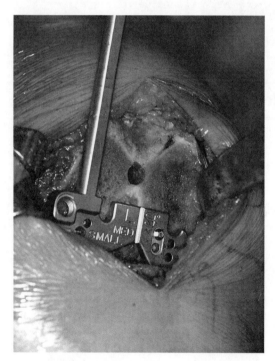

Fig. 11.9 Distal femoral sizing guide is initially placed under the femoral condyle in flexion. This is aligned with *Whitesides line*

positioned, it is fixed to the distal femur with two pins. The knee is then placed in extension and the femoral sizing guide is then attached to the anterior sizing rod. The anterior referencing finger is placed on the anterior lateral surface of the anterior femur, and adjusted to avoid anterior femoral notching (Fig. 11.10). The size of the femur is read from the femoral sizing guide. Usually, when between sizes, the smaller size is chosen for cruciate-retaining knees while the larger size is chosen for the posterior-stabilized knees (Fig. 11.10). The anterior reference finger is removed. With the knee flexed to 80–90°, the drill guide is positioned in the slot where the anterior reference finger was removed. With this guide, two drill holes are placed in the distal femur, which creates the reference for the final femoral finishing guide.

With the knee still flexed to 80–90°, the proper femoral finishing guide is then placed under the patella on the distal femur. Two pins are placed through the femoral finishing guide in the drill holes in the distal femur. The knee is then positioned in full extension and the femoral finishing guide is then positioned centrally on the femur. In this extended position, both the lateral and medial edges of the femoral condyles are easily seen. In extension, a medial screw pin is used to fix the guide to the femur. The knee is then flexed to 40° so that the lateral screw can be placed. Retractors are then positioned around the collateral ligaments. The femoral finishing guide is used to complete the final femoral cuts (Fig. 11.11). The femoral finishing guide is then removed and the resected femoral cuts are removed (Fig. 11.12).

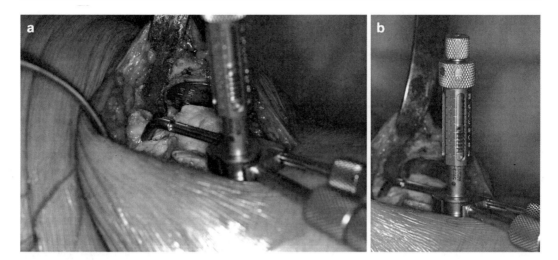

Fig. 11.10 Distal femoral sizing guide. (**a**) Anterior view after attachment of the anterior referencing arm. (**b**) Sizing guide is shown. The sizing shown here is between "*D*" and "*E*." In this cruciate-retaining TKA, a size "*D*" is chosen

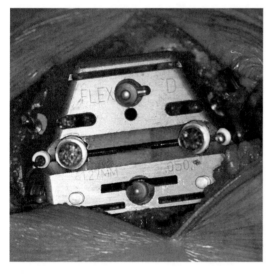

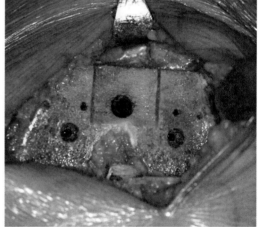

Fig. 11.12 The distal femur finished

Fig. 11.11 Femoral finishing guide on the distal femur

Testing the Components

First the knee is placed in extension with retractors around the tibia. The tibia is sized in extension where the entire surface can be seen. Then the knee is placed in 90° of flexion, with Hohmann retractors positioned over the medial and lateral femoral condyles. The femoral trial component is then positioned between these retractors and maneuvered onto the distal femur. Care is taken to align the femoral trial with the lug holes before final seating of the trial. The knee is again extended to take tension off the extensor mechanism and the tibial trial is positioned with the tibial insert. Stability and range of motion is then assessed and any adjustments are made, as with a standard technique. The trial tibial tray is then pinned in place with the knee in extension. The tibial insert is removed in extension and the knee is flexed to remove the trial femoral component. In this flexed positioned,

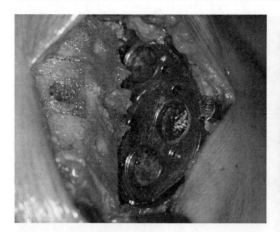

Fig. 11.13 Preparation of the tibia for the four-pegged component

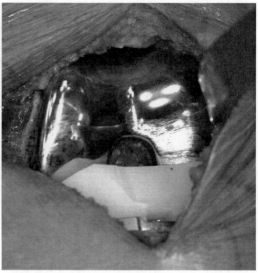

Fig. 11.15 Final components in place

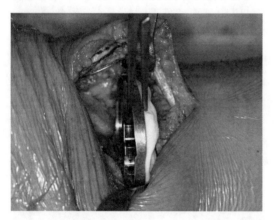

Fig. 11.14 Cementing of the tibial component in extension. This allows the tibia to be completely visualized and excess cement removed

the tibia is prepared for the four-pegged tibial component by drilling the four pegs (Fig. 11.13).

Fixation of Final Components

A cemented or porous ingrowth femoral component may be used. The tibial and patellar components are fixed with cement. In extension, the tibia is irrigated and a layer of cement is placed on the tibial plateau with an angled nozzle cement gun and cement is also placed on the back of the tibial component. The tibial component is then placed on the tibial plateau (Fig. 11.14).

The component is compressed against the tibia, starting posterior-laterally and progressing anterior-medially; this extrudes cement anterior-medially, where it is easy to remove. A spacer block is used to place pressure on the tibial component in extension while extruded cement is removed from the posterior and peripheral component with a series of cement removal curettes. The cement on the tibia is allowed to fully cure to avoid tibial component shift during femoral component placement.

If a cemented femur is used, meticulous removal of cement must be completed. A porous ingrowth femoral component obviates cement removal. The knee is placed in 90° of flexion with Hohmann retractors positioned over the medial and lateral femoral condyles. The femoral component is then positioned between these retractors and maneuvered onto the distal femur. Care is taken to align the femoral component with the lug holes before final seating of the component. The knee is again extended to take tension off the extensor mechanism and a polyethylene spacer is inserted into place with the knee at 15° of flexion with traction on the tibia (Fig. 11.15). Finally, the patella is cemented with second batch of cement. Stability and range

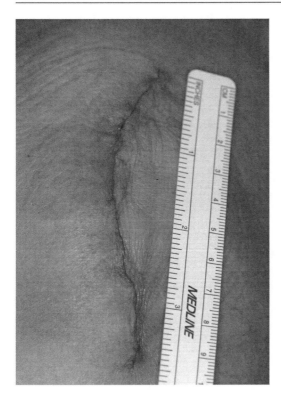

Fig. 11.16 Skin after wound closure is complete

of motion is then assessed and any adjustments are made as with a standard technique.

Wound Closure

The knee is irrigated and a drain is placed. The retinaculum is closed with #1 Vicryl sutures. The deep layer of adipose and the dermis are closed with 2–0 Vicryl. A running 3–0 Monocryl and Dermabond are used to close and seal the skin (Fig. 11.16).

Conclusion

TKA with the quadriceps-sparing approach avoids violation of the quadriceps tendon, VMO fibers, and subvastus interval. In addition, since the interval remains in the retinaculum, the incision cannot self-extend with retraction as the subvastus and midvastus approaches. Furthermore, along with rapid perioperative recovery protocols [2],

patients usually ambulate with minimal assistance and are discharged to home later on the same day of surgery [3].

This minimally invasive approach to total knee replacement is very safe. Furthermore, this approach potential can be easily extended into a medial parapatellar or midvastus approach if needed. Converse to the traditional approach to total knee replacement, where the hyperflexion of the knee increases exposure, extension improves exposure in this quadriceps-sparing approach. Lastly, this technique cannot be completed with traditional cutting guides; proper retractors and cutting guides are necessary to complete each step in this procedure.

References

1. Berger RA, Deirmengian CA, Della Valle CJ, Paprosky WG, Jacobs JJ, Rosenberg AG. A technique for minimally invasive, quadriceps-sparing total knee arthroplasty. *J Knee Surg*, 19(1):63–70, 2006
2. Berger RA, Sanders S, D'Ambrogio E, Buchheit K, Deirmengian C, Paprosky W, Della Valle CJ, Rosenberg AG. Minimally invasive quadriceps-sparing TKA: results of a comprehensive pathway for outpatient TKA. *J Knee Surg*, 19(2):145–148, 2006
3. Berger RA, Sanders S, Gerlinger T, Della Valle C, Jacobs JJ, Rosenberg AG. Outpatient total knee arthroplasty with a minimally invasive technique. *J Arthroplasty*, 20(6 Suppl 3):33–38, 2005
4. Bonutti PM, Mont MA, McMahon M, Ragland PS, Kester M. Minimally invasive total knee arthroplasty. *J Bone Joint Surg Am*, 86-A(Suppl 2):26–32, 2004
5. Goble EM, Justin DF. Minimally invasive total knee replacement: principles and technique. *Orthop Clin North Am*, 35(2):235–245, 2004
6. Hofmann AA, Plaster RL, Murdock LE. Subvastus (Southern) approach for primary total knee arthroplasty. *Clin Orthop Relat Res*, (269):70–77, 1991
7. Laskin RS. Minimally invasive total knee replacement using a mini-mid vastus incision technique and results. *Surg Technol Int*, 13:231–238, 2004
8. Laskin RS, Beksac B, Phongjunakorn A, Pittors K, Davis J, Shim JC, Pavlov H, Petersen M. Minimally invasive total knee replacement through a mini-midvastus incision: an outcome study. *Clin Orthop Relat Res*, (428):74–81, 2004
9. Tria AJ, Jr. Minimally invasive total knee arthroplasty: the importance of instrumentation. *Orthop Clin North Am*, 35(2):227–234, 2004
10. Tria AJ, Jr, Coon TM. Minimal incision total knee arthroplasty: early experience. *Clin Orthop Relat Res*, (416):185–190, 2003

Bi-unicompartmental Knee Protheses

12

Sergio Romagnoli, Francesco Verde, Eddie Bibbiani, Nicolò Castelnuovo, and F. d'Amario

In the past few years, with the introduction of minimally invasive surgery (MIS) and based on excellent unicompartmental prosthesis (UKR) long-term results, we are experiencing a renewed interest in single or associate compartmental substitutions of the knee compared with anterior cruciate ligament (ACL). The UKR prosthesis is used in tissue-sparing surgeries (TSS) [1]. TSS is a surgical philosophy that mandates a maximum respect for tissues and for anatomy and biomechanics. The aim of TSS is to reduce aggressive local and general surgical procedures, and thereby to optimize the patient's postoperative course and functional recovery. The surgical access routes in TSS are chosen with respect to the soft tissues, cartilaginous tissue, and bones. Surgical incision of the skin, a soft tissue, is minimized as much as possible while still permitting the intervention and the correct implantation of the prosthesis. The surgery is performed with care taken for the blood vessels and nerves, but also for the musculotendinous apparatus and the capsuloligamentous system.

The use of unicompartmental prostheses in the knee, especially those that require only minimal bone removal, represent a fundamental use for TSS. These unicompartmental prostheses have led, almost automatically, to the use of small, conservative access routes. Even more than in the hip, uni-

compartmental knee prostheses require careful insertion into the complex biomechanical and kinematic situation of the knee, especially when bi-unicompartmental prostheses are used. In this case, the tissue-sparing principal that the prosthesis does not substitute for the joint but integrates with it is especially apparent. In fact, when implanting a UKR, it is wrong to correct the joint biomechanics that caused the pathology; instead, one simply substitutes the part that degenerated due to the disease.

Bicompartmental prosthesis was introduced in the 1970s by Marmor, Gunston, and Lubinus [2, 3]. The surgical technique is based on the substitution of the two femorotibial compartments using two femoral and two tibial independent components preserving the tibial eminentia and the ACL. With the term *bicompartmental*, we mean a surgical procedure that substitutes one only of the tibiofemoral compartments in association with the patellofemoral (PF) compartment. Actually, the improved screening technique and treatment of knee arthritis enable more young patients to consider prosthetic surgery. In these cases, minimally invasive conservative solutions are sought that can guarantee maximum results to patients with high-level expectations.

Epidemiology

In the treatment of bicompartmental arthritis, the presence of a functional ACL represents the basis of the surgical indication. In the last 1,000 bi-tricompartmental implants performed at the Centro

S. Romagnoli (✉) • F. Verde • E. Bibbiani
• N. Castelnuovo • F. d'Amario
Centro Chirurgia Protesica, Istituto Ortopedico
"R. Galeazzi,", Milan, Italy
e-mail: sergio.romagnoli@gruppsandonato.it

di Chirurgia Protesica at the Istituto Ortopedico Galeazzi in Milano, we have observed that, in 35.1% of the cases, the patients had an intact ACL, while in 15.7% of cases, the ACL appeared slightly degenerated but still functioning, and finally, in 49.2% of cases, the ACL could not be observed intraoperatively. We studied the relationship between the ACL and its mechanical function in a long-term survivorship study of bicompartmental prosthesis and in the Allegretto (Zimmer) unicompartmental prosthesis with 10–15 years of follow-up [4–12]. This article and several other long-term survivorship studies of unicompartmental prosthesis [6–16] show that anteroposterior (AP) long-term stability remains unchanged. This shows that the ACL has the ability to maintain the same mechanical function over the course of years. As a matter of fact, in our studies on 124 patients treated with unicompartmental prosthesis, we had only one case of failure due to ACL deficiency.

If we consider age as a selective criteria, we observe that in 1,000 cases of knee prosthesis performed, 7.6% of patients were younger than 55 years of age while 25.8% were aged between 55 and 65 years, 39.5% were aged between 65 and 75 years, and 27.1% were older than 75 years of age. Therefore, 33.4% of patients were younger than 65 years of age. Thirty-five percent of these patients had an intact ACL and were potential users of cruciate-retaining prostheses.

Indications

This surgery is indicated for patients with bilateral femorotibial degeneration but with an asymptomatic patella, with cruciate ligament integrity, flexum deformity <5°, varus-valgus deformity <15°, and range of motion (ROM) >80° (Fig. 12.1) [8, 9, 13].

Radiographic evaluation is based on AP, lateral, and sky view projections that show a femorotibial degeneration higher than grade I on Ahlback scale and a PF involvement lower than grade II. Furthermore, on a long weight-bearing AP X-ray view, we can calculate the mechanical axis of the limb, highlighting the correct range of tolerated deformity. Magnetic resonance imaging (MRI) can highlight both an ACL instability or deficiency and

a PF degeneration. The knee must be stable clinically, and only a minimal laxity due to cartilaginous degeneration is tolerated. We can usually observe clinical signs, such as pain while walking and climbing stairs and effusion. Age and weight are not a limit, but this solution is especially suitable in active patients younger than 65 years of age and with a body mass index (BMI) < 32. Bi-Uni is, in fact, suitable in young patients with high functional expectations. As previously mentioned, the main limits of this implantation selection are ACL and PF integrity. In the first case, when a femorotibial bicompartmental degeneration defines a correct indication for a Bi-Uni implant, but the absence of ACL is a clear limitation, only then can we consider an ACL reconstruction.

A secondary degeneration of PF joint with chronic anterior pain is something to keep in mind when selecting patients. Evaluation criteria are symptoms, X-ray evaluation of alignment and overload, and the intraoperative evidence of grade III or IV chondromalacia. Symptoms, only if accompanied by other parameters, which can be X-ray or intraoperative observation, are a clear limit to the indication. Bi-UKR can sometimes be the result of a UKR revision due to degeneration and the pain of the untreated femorotibial compartment. In this case, the implant of a UKR in the other degenerated compartment of the same knee results in a Bi-UKR. Obviously, in this case, the previous implant must be stable, and the only contraindications are polyethylene (PE) wear and ACL deficiency (Fig. 12.2). Absolute contraindications to the Bi-UKR are ligaments instability, severe axial deformity >15°, flexum deformity >5°, and compartmental bone stock defect >12 mm.

Surgical Technique

Bi-UKR uses the same surgical technique as UKR applied to both the medial and lateral compartments. We can choose between two different approaches: a double mini skin incision or an isolated medial parapatellar approach. The first choice relies on a parapatellar medial, 4- to 6-cm mini skin incision and a mini lateral parapatellar incision of 6–8 cm, depending on the individual case. Usually, we start in the medial compartment with

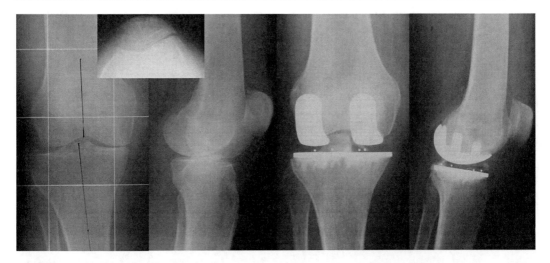

Fig. 12.1 Bicompartmental knee arthritis with asymptomatic and not degenerated PF joint (56-year-old woman)

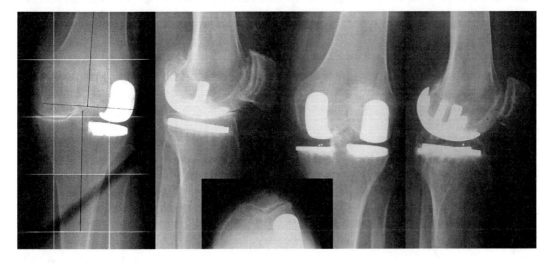

Fig. 12.2 Medial UKR, compatible with the existing UKR (16 years follow-up), due to medial compartment degeneration

a tibia-first technique; once we have positioned the trials, we proceed with cutting the lateral compartment. This gives us the perception of the stability we want to reach. The second choice, which we prefer, is based on a minimally invasive parapatellar medial incision of 8–10 cm. In this case, a mini-midvastus incision allows patella subluxation, creating a good exposition of both the medial and lateral compartments. Once the compartments are exposed, surface bone cuts are performed with the tibia-first technique. Tibial cuts are performed using a minimally invasive tibial guide at the same time in the two compartments. Vertical cuts have to be between 15 and 20° oblique on the AP axis of the medial compartment and 10–15° in the lateral,

respecting the ACL [9]. The horizontal cut must respect the height and obliquity of the joint line, reproducing the perpendicular cut more on the proximal epiphysary axis than on the diaphysary axis (Fig. 12.3).

The obliquity of the joint line varies depending on the varus or valgus morphotype and so allows us to avoid the need for a release. In the sagittal plane, the tibial cut must reproduce the preoperative slope and respect posterior cruciate ligament (PCL) integrity. On the femoral side, we perform the distal cut in extension and the posterior cut in flexion using a tensor guide that calibrates the same amount of resections, creating a balanced flexion-extension gap (Fig. 12.4).

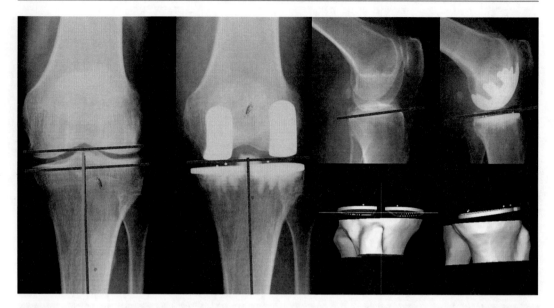

Fig. 12.3 Obliquity and slope joint line respect

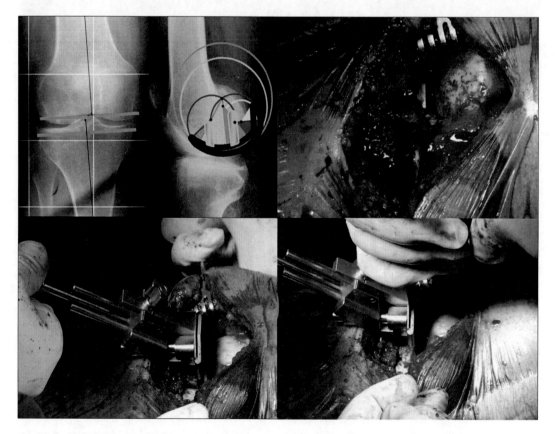

Fig. 12.4 Femoral distal curt in extension with tensor guide and spacer in the opposite compartment

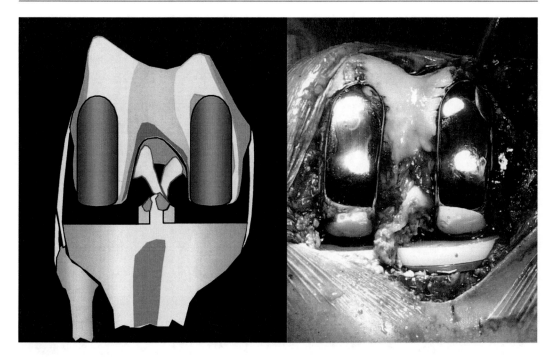

Fig. 12.5 Component lateralization

First, the distal cut in extension creates the perception of the stability we want to reach, adjusting the tensor to avoid overcorrection and release. Subsequently, the flexion cut is calibrated on the same quantity and tension in order to obtain balance. The same thickness of the prosthesis to be implanted needs to be removed (2 mm), 2–3 mm of bone from the medial femoral condyle and 1–2 mm from the lateral, depending on the axis correction needed. Femoral components are often lateralized to obtain a femorotibial centralization in flexion-extension (Fig. 12.5). Once we have assessed the stability with the trials, we prepare the bone for cementing (Fig. 12.6).

In well-selected cases of young patients in whom the only limit to Bi-UKR is the absence of the ACL, we can perform a reconstruction procedure (Fig. 12.7). Currently, we prefer using hamstrings to avoid complications caused by patellar tendons. In this case, tibial fixation is done right before femoral cementing. In young patients, in whom PF joints are symptomatic, together with grade II-III chondromalacia observed intraoperatively, we use a bicondylar femoral component with an ACL-retention design. Actually, a cruciate-retaining total knee arthroplasty (TKA) is another interesting solution, but is more invasive (Fig. 12.8).

Complications

Bicompartmental implant failure may be caused by intraoperative complications or it may occur over time. Intraoperative complications include incorrect positioning of components, tibial eminentia fracture, incorrect ligament balancing, and cementation mistakes. In the case of tibial eminentia fracture during surgery, this can be stabilized with one or two divergent cortical screws that have to be fixed before cementation [9–13] (Fig. 12.9).

Long-term follow-up in cases treated with eminentia fixation have never shown secondary loosening of the intercondylar spine. Complications that occurred over the course of time included PF joint degeneration or secondary ligament degeneration, component loosening, or PE wear. Finally, septic loosening has the same incidence as in other prosthetic procedures.

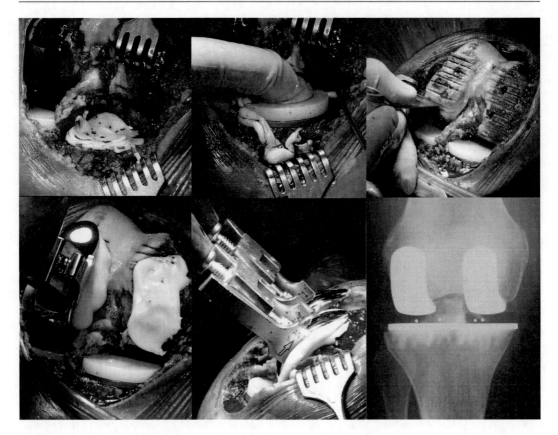

Fig. 12.6 Surgical technique and cementation of tibia and femur. We start with lateral tibial compartment cementation

Bicompartmental Arthritis

Knee arthritis often involves only one of the two femorotibial compartments, along with symptomatic PF joint degeneration. Among our patients, this represents only 15% of knee arthritis, whereas 5% have isolated bicompartmental femorotibial involvement. Treatment of bicompartmental arthritis involves a lateral or medial UKR to treat arthritis and correct the axial deformity and the use of a PF prosthesis [14]. This combined use widens indications and reduces limits to a UKR and isolated PF prosthesis. This procedure is suitable in cases of borderline UKR indications with femorotibial compartmental arthritis and symptomatic patella and in cases of borderline indications for PF prosthesis due to isolated PF arthritis with 3° mechanical axis deviation and initial femorotibial unicompartmental involvement.

In our experience, two kinds of bicompartmental arthritis exist, femorotibial and PF. In the first case, an initial PF joint pathology is associated with an axial limb deviation, with varus or valgus morphotype and secondary femorotibial arthritis. In the second case, the pathology initially concerns one of the two femorotibial compartments with a varus or valgus morphotype involving the secondary PF joint. The isolated use of the isolated PF prosthesis is an uncommon procedure with few references in the literature and even rarer is the combined use with a UKR. The advantages of a bicompartmental implant, UKR plus PF, are cruciate preservation, respect for rotational axis, bone stock preservation, patellar height and tracking, normal joint kinematic reproduction, and morphotype respect. Selection criteria are the same as for UKR in which the PF joint is degenerated (Fig. 12.10).

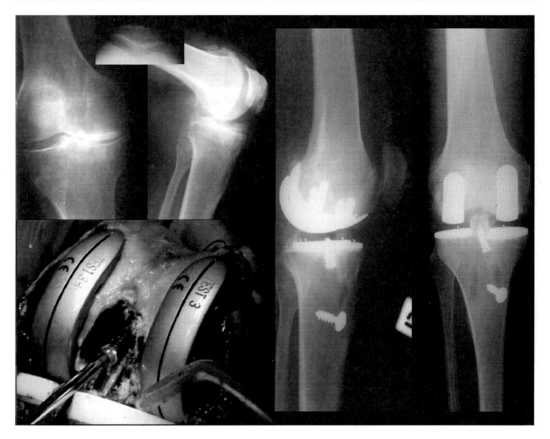

Fig. 12.7 A 53-year-old man with a bilateral meniscectomy and ACL rupture sequelae. A BTB reconstruction procedure was performed in 1998

The surgical approach is the same as in UKR, medial in varus or lateral in valgus, but 2–3 cm longer [4, 8, 10, 12]. Usually, the procedure starts with UKR steps, the tibia-first technique, and a distal femoral cut in extension. Once stability has been tested with trials, continue with the preparation of the implant surface for the PF prosthesis, first the femoral trochlea and then the patella. It is important to keep a distance of >3 mm between the two prosthetic components. Our objective is to respect the femoral surfaces rotational axis and trochlear depth, avoiding excessive tension on the patella. Trials implanted must highlight perfect PF tracking without patellar clunk and tilting in the area of the component transition.

Biomechanics

Preserving both cruciate ligaments in unicondylar knee arthroplasty provides more normal knee mechanic function, and it contributes to enhanced patient function as shown in our study in 2001 [11]. Preserving both cruciate ligaments with total knee arthroplasty should provide functional benefit if compared with arthroplasty, which sacrifices one or both cruciate ligaments. We have compared knee kinematics in patients with well-functioning cruciate-preserving medial unicondylar and bi-unicondylar arthroplasty to determine if knee motions were different.

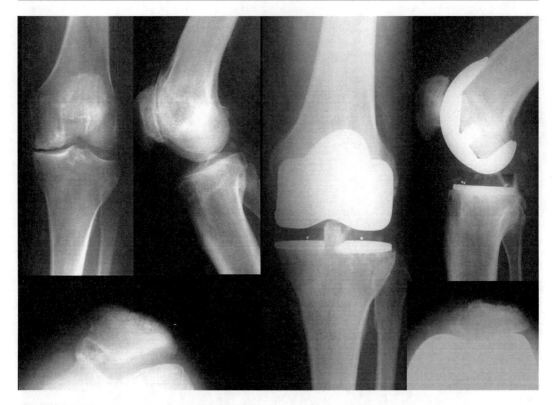

Fig. 12.8 Bi-UKR with total femur (NexGen CR, Zimmer) in the case of symptomatic PF degeneration

Material and Methods

Twelve consenting patients with seven medial unicondylar and five bi-unicondylar arthroplasties participated in this Institutional Review Board-approved study (Table 12.1). Patients were recruited for participation based on combined Knee Society scores greater than 195 [17] at a minimum of 8 months after surgery, who returned to high levels of activity after arthroplasty, had high satisfaction with the procedure and outcome, and had a willingness to drive up to 4 h to participate in the study. All patients had surgery by a single surgeon (SR) using a cemented metal-backed fixed-bearing tibial baseplate and a cemented cobalt-chrome femoral prosthesis (Allegretto, Centerpulse Orthopedics Ltd., Winterthur, Switzerland). The surgical technique fully maintained both cruciate ligaments and replicated as closely as possible the normal articular surfaces and posterior slope of each tibial plateau. Tibial prostheses were implanted in 2–3° varus with respect to the tibial mechanical axis. Femoral prostheses were positioned perpendicular to the tibial implants with resurfacing bone preparation. The medial and lateral femoral components were lateralized slightly to maintain contact on the center of the tibial bearing surface with flexion and endorotation/exorotation. Patients' knee motions were recorded using lateral fluoroscopy during treadmill gait at 1 m/s, single limb stepping up and down on a 25-cm stair, maximum flexion in a lunge with the foot placed on the 25-cm step, maximum flexion kneeling on a padded stool, and weight-bearing straight-leg stance.

Image matching-based measurements of knee arthroplasty kinematics typically use surface models of the implanted metal components.

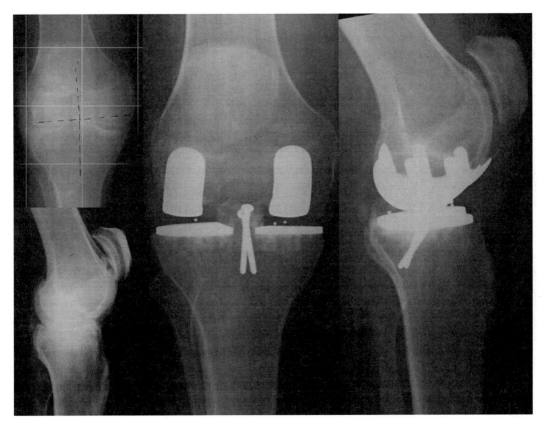

Fig. 12.9 Fixation of intraoperative tibial eminentia fracture with two divergent cortical screws

Since the tibial components of this unicondylar system had only a thin metal wafer base and two small beads within the PE, it was determined that a shape model incorporating implant and bone geometry would permit better measurement sensitivity and robustness for large out-of-plane motions. The three-dimensional position and orientation of the proximal and distal knee segments was determined using a toolbox of model-based shape-matching techniques, including previously reported techniques [24], manual matching, and automated matching using non-linear least-squares (modified Levenberg-Marquardt) techniques (Fig. 12.11).

Three thousand two hundred and eleven fluoroscopic images, an average of 268 images per knee, were analyzed. The results of this shape-matching process have standard errors of approximately $0.5–1.0°$ for rotations and $0.5–1.0$ mm for translations in the sagittal plane [18]. Joint kinematics were determined from the three-dimensional pose of each knee component using Cardan/Euler angles [19]. The anterior/posterior locations of tibiofemoral contact were computed, independently for each implanted compartment, by transforming the joint pose into a reference system parallel to the transverse plane of the flat tibial component and finding the lowest point on the femoral component. For the stair, kneeling, and lunge activities, kinematics were expressed relative to the joint pose in straight-leg weight-bearing stance. For gait, the kinematics were expressed relative to the joint pose at heel-strike. Kneeling and lunge data were compared using t-tests. For the stair and gait data, an average curve for each knee was created from four trials of data. These average curves were then combined to create group averages.

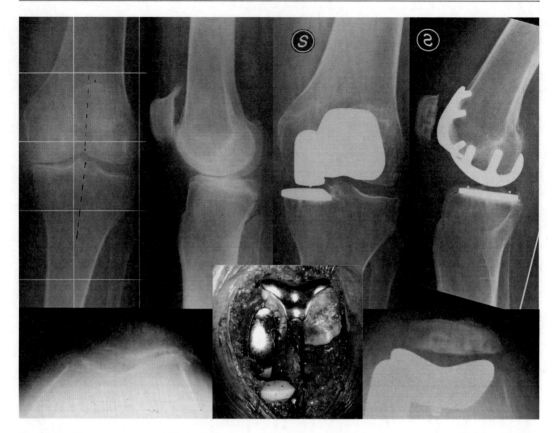

Fig. 12.10 Bicompartmental arthritis (medial compartment plus PF) and solution with a combined PF+UKR implant

Table 12.1 Characteristics of knee replacement patients

Sex	Age (year)	Weight (kg)	Right knee	Right follow-up (months)	Left knee	Left follow-up (months)	Lifestyle
M	42	75	Healthy		Bi-Uni	26	Sports
F	55	65	Bi-Uni	18	Healthy		Active
F	60	80	Bi-Uni[a]	8	Uni	9	Long walk
M	73	78	Uni	10	Uni	10	Long walk
M	73	75	Bi-Uni	21	Healthy		Sports
M	74	72	Uni	21	Uni	21	Sports
F	79	74	Uni	15	Uni	22	Long walk
M	79	65	Uni[b]		Bi-uni	36	Active

From [11]

[a] Total knee replacement femoral component used with bi-unicondylar tibial components

[b] Well-functioning unicondylar knee, but no computed tomography (CT) data to permit inclusion in study

Results

Maximum knee flexion in kneeling and lunge was an average of 10° greater ($P>0.22$) for unicondylar knees at 135°/133° (Table 12.2). Average tibial internal rotation was greater in the unicondylar knees for kneeling ($P=0.18$) and lunge ($P=0.06$) activities. None of these differences was statistically significant. Posterior translation of the medial condyle averaged 2 mm or less for both

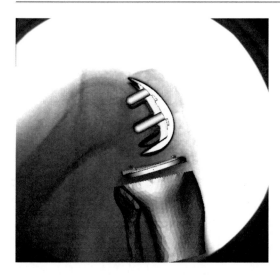

Fig. 12.11 Three-dimensional pose measurements for the femur and tibia/fibula segments were accomplished by projecting the shape models onto the digitized and distortion-corrected fluoroscopic images. The model pose was varied until the projected shapes matched those in the image

types of knees in the lunge and kneeling activities. Posterior translation of the lateral condyle in the bi-unicondylar knees averaged 4 mm for the lunge and kneeling activities. Both groups of knees showed tibial internal rotation with flexion during the stair activity (Fig. 12.12).

The unicondylar knees showed greater tibial rotation for flexion from 20 to 80° ($P < 0.01$). For 0–30° flexion during the stair activity, the medial condyle translated posterior 3.5 ± 2.5 mm in unicondylar knees and 4.7 ± 1.9 mm in bi-unicondylar knees ($P = 0.035$). Lateral condyle posterior translation was 5.0 ± 2.3 mm in bi-unicondylar knees for 0–30° flexion. The bi-unicondylar knees showed greater knee flexion from heel-strike to midstance phase than the unicondylar knees ($P < 0.01$), but similar flexion from late stance through swing phase (Fig. 12.13a). The bi-unicondylar knees showed greater tibial external rotation throughout stance phase ($P < 0.01$; Fig. 12.13b), which correlates closely to greater posterior translation of the medial condyle in early to mid stance phase ($P < 0.01$, Fig. 12.13c). Lateral condylar AP translations in the bi-unicondylar knees were

similar in pattern, but smaller in magnitude, compared with the medial condylar translations (Fig. 12.13d).

Discussion

Well-done contemporary knee arthroplasty provides excellent 10-year outcomes almost without regard to the particular philosophy or implant type used. In this context, the focus for improvement shifts to patients' functional abilities and limitations. Contemporary unicondylar knee arthroplasty is widely acknowledged to provide more normal postoperative function compared with total knee arthroplasty, and it is assumed that retaining both cruciate ligaments contributes to this functional advantage. It is natural, therefore, to ask whether bi-unicondylar knee arthroplasty might provide similar knee kinematics and function. This study attempts to answer that question for a highly selected small group of active patients with excellent outcomes. This selected group of unicondylar and bi-unicondylar knees showed average maximum flexion that was equivalent to or better than has been previously reported for knee arthroplasty in Western patients [20–23]. These knees prove that excellent flexion can be achieved with these techniques, but it is likely that the mean maximum flexion would be less for a more broadly representative group of patients. Kinematics in both groups varied substantially between knees for the deep flexion activities, so that no statistically significant differences could be demonstrated (Table 12.2). Posterior translation of the medial condyle with flexion was observed in both knee groups for the stair activity, 3.5 mm for the unicondylar and 5 mm for the bi-unicondylar knees. This finding is consistent with prior studies of anterior cruciate ligament-retaining total knee arthroplasty [24, 25], but the translations were greater than reported in studies of medial unicondylar knee arthroplasty [26] or the healthy knee [23, 27] for quasistatic activities. It was particularly surprising in the bi-unicondylar knees that the medial and lateral condyles translated posteriorly the same amount in early flexion (0–40°), again contrasting with reports for normal knee

Table 12.2 Knee kinematics in deep flexion kneeling and lunge postures (mean ± 1 standard deviation, range in parentheses)

Parameter	Kneeling		Lunge	
	Uni	Bi-Uni	Uni	Bi-Uni
Flexion (degrees)	135 ± 14 (114–150)	123 ± 14 (108–136)	133 ± 15 (111–150)	124 ± 12 (107–135)
Axial rotation (degrees)	9.0 ± 6 (3–19)	3 ± 7 (−3–13)	12.0 ± 7 (−1–19)	4 ± 6 (−2–12)
Medial rollback (mm)	2 ± 5 (−5–11)	0 ± 5 (−6–5)	2 ± 4 (−2–11)	1 ± 5 (−6–6)
Lateral rollback (mm)		4 ± 9 (−4–16)		3 ± 9 (−6–16)

From [11]

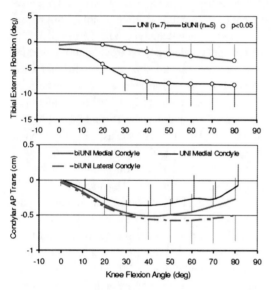

Fig. 12.12 The pattern of tibial rotation (mean ± 1 standard deviation) for Uni and Bi-Uni knees differed (*P* < 0.001) during the stair activity (*top*). Medial condyle AP translations also differed (*P* = 0.035), but there were no statistically significant differences for specific flexion ranges (*bottom*). AP translations for the medial and lateral condyles of the Bi-Uni knees were the same from 0 to 40° flexion. The *white circles* indicate where there is a significant pair-wise difference between the two data series (From [11]. with kind permission of Springer Science+Business Media)

kinematics during quasistatic activities [23, 28]. The unicondylar knees showed less than 2 mm AP translation of the medial condyle during the stance phase of gait. The bi-unicondylar knees showed more than 5 mm posterior translation of the medial condyle just after heel-strike, indicating greater dynamic laxity. Two factors likely contributed to increased medial condylar sliding. First, these knees had greater flexion in early

stance phase, so the knees were in a position of increased passive laxity [28].

Second, the bi-unicondylar knees had bicompartmental disease preoperatively and no longer maintained the normal laxity of the lateral compartment after arthroplasty. As a result, the pattern of motion during gait in the bi-unicondylar knees was closer to motions reported for fixed-bearing total knee replacements in identical tests [28, 29]. As reported by others and confirmed in this study, preserving both cruciate ligaments in knee arthroplasty maintains some basic features of normal knee kinematics, including posterior translation of the femoral condyles and tibial internal rotation with flexion. These motions were most evident during the stair activity for the unicondylar and bi-unicondylar knees. As one might expect, the dynamic laxity of the knee increased when both tibiofemoral compartments were replaced, which was most apparent during gait. In conclusion, the kinematics of unicondylar and bi-unicondylar knee arthroplasty share common features, but differ in ways that are consistent with bicompartmental preoperative disease and loss of the normal lateral compartment in the bi-unicondylar knees. Despite kinematic differences compared with unicondylar knees, bi-unicondylar arthroplasty can provide functional outcomes similar to unicondylar knees in appropriately selected patients.

Results

We started our experience in 1990 and until now, the percentage of Bi-UKR has been modified each year. However, from 1990 to 2006, the percentage of Bi-UKR was 2.3%, while from July

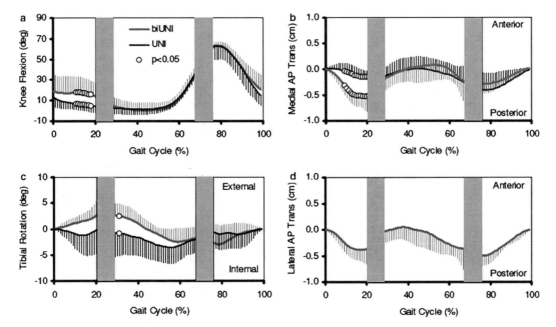

Fig. 12.13 Knee kinematics during gait differed between the Uni and Bi-Uni knees (mean ± 1 standard deviation). The Bi-Uni knees showed greater flexion in early stance, but similar flexion in late stance and swing (**a**) Bi-Uni knees showed greater tibial external rotation during stance (**b**) Bi-Uni knees showed significantly greater posterior translations of the medial condyle in early stance (**c**), and a similar pattern of AP motion for the lateral condyle (**d**). The two *gray regions* on each graph indicate gaps in the fluoroscopic data, when the contralateral knee occludes the view, which are filled by interpolation. The *white circles* indicate where there is a significant pair-wise difference between the two data series (From [11]. with kind permission of Springer Science + Business Media)

2002 to 2006 it was 4.8%; however, if we consider only patients younger than 55 years, from 1990 to 2006 the percentage was 14.6%. This confirms that this surgical option is strongly indicated in young active patients. The UKR + PF, bicompartmental implants, performed from 2003 to 2005 represent 8% of our knee implants. This surgical technique, which seems new, is actually the result of 15 years of experience, during which, the indications were restricted to isolated PF knee arthritis and to surgical treatment of unicompartmental knee arthroplasty for chronic anterior knee pain due to secondary PF degeneration. In 2006 we revised our three main types of implants related to ACL: Bi-UKR with two femoral and tibial independent components, Bi-UKR with two tibial components and a total femoral component and ACL retaining, and bicompartmental UKR + PF (we have always used Allegretto, Zimmer unicompartmental prosthesis, with tibia Sulmesh and minimum PE thickness of 6 mm). From 1990 to 2005, we performed 148 Bi-UKR

and 103 with two independent tibial components and that were total femur and ACL retaining (Fig. 12.14). We have studied 129 Bi-UKR consecutive cases with independent femoral components implanted between 1990 and 2005 with a 1- to 15-year follow-up. This study has proved a medium ROM of 126°. In this series, we had three failures, one caused by acquired ligament instability, another caused by PF degeneration, and the last one for chronic anterior knee pain.

We have also studied 91 consecutive cases of prosthesis with tibia bicompartmental and total femur implanted between 1990 and 2003 with 2- to 11 -year follow-up. In this series, the average ROM was 116° and we had one failure due to ligament instability. In 88 cases of bicompartmental prosthesis (UKR + PF) 3 years after the indication extension, we had only one case of failure due to patellar tilt related to prosthetic design, which we eventually abandoned, and revision with a primary total knee implant (Fig. 12.15).

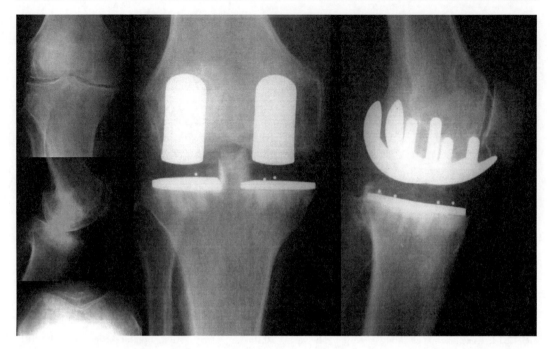

Fig. 12.14 Radiographs showing 12-year follow-up after Bi-Uni

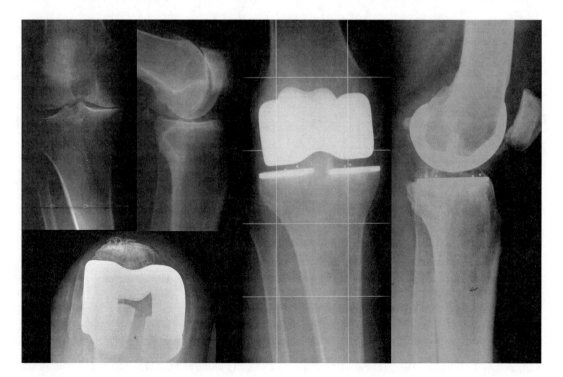

Fig. 12.15 Radiographs showing 11-year follow-up after Bi-UKR with total femur

Conclusion

The cruciate-retaining knee bicompartmental arthroplasties, even if not common, seem to offer a high level functionality and a joint kinematic that presents essential features similar to a normal knee and a survivor rate comparable to TKA. Bi-UKR has shown an average range of motion of 126°, higher than the average standard total knee replacement (TKR). Bi-UKR with total femur has never used a resurfaced patella, but despite this has never shown PF long-term complications. UKR + PF represent the technique's further expansion with good prospects for the future.

References

1. Pipino F (2006) Tissue sparing surgery (T.S.S.) in hip and knee arthroplasty. J Orthop Traumatol 7:33–35
2. Gunston FH (1971) Polycentric knee arthroplasty. Prosthetic simulation of normal knee movement. J Bone Joint Surg Br 53(2):272–277
3. Marmor L (1973) The modular knee. Clin Orthop Relat Res 94:242–248
4. Romagnoli S, Verde F, Eberle RW (2006) 10-year minimum follow-up of medial unicompartmental knee arthroplasty with the allegretto prosthesis. Presented at AAOS, Chicago 2006, San Francisco 2007; exhibit SE41, Poster P203
5. Romagnoli S (1996) The unicompartmental knee prosthesis and the rotatory gonarthrosis kinematic. In: Current Concept in Primary and Revision, Total Knee Arthroplasty, edited by John N. Insall, W. Norman Scott, Giles R. Scuderi, Lippincott-Raven Publishers, Philadelphia
6. Cartier P, Sanouiller JL, Grelsamer RP (1996) Unicompartmental knee arthroplasty surgery. 10 years minimum follow-up period. J Arthroplasty 11(7):782–788
7. Romagnoli S, Grappiolo G, Ursino N, Broch C (2000) Dexa evaluation of bone remodelling in the proximal tibial after unicompartmental prosthesis. Traumalinc 2:2 Pabst Science Publishers
8. Romagnoli S, Grappiolo G, Camera A (1998) Indicazioni e limiti delle protesi monocompartimentali, Il Ginocchio, Anno XIV, vol. 18
9. Romagnoli S, Camera A, Bertolotti M, Arnaldi E (2000) La protesi Bimonocompartimentale con rispetto ricostruzione del LCA, Il Ginocchio, Anno XIV, vol. 19, anno
10. Romagnoli S, Camera A, Bertolotti M (2000) Deformità rotatoria e protesi monocompartimentale, Il Ginocchio, Anno XVI, vol. 19
11. Romagnoli S, Banks SA, Fregly BJ, Boniforti F, Reinschmidt C (2005) Comparing in vivo kinematics of unicondylar and bi-unicondylar knee replacement. Knee Surg Sports Traumatol Arthrosc 13(7):551–6
12. Romagnoli S (2004) Allegretto: Protesi Monocompartimentale di ginocchio. Pronews, Anno 2 – numero 1, Marzo
13. "Die unicondylare Schlittenprothese – (Unicompartmental Knee Arthroplasty). Klaus Buckup Herausgeber, Steinkopff Darmstadt 2005
14. "Bi-Unikondylare Schlittenprothese" S. Romagnoli, F.Verde
15. Romagnoli S., Verde F., Damario F., Castelnuovo N (2006) La protesi femoro-rotulea. Archivio di Ortopedia e Traumatologia 117(1)-
16. Chassin EP, Mikosz RP, Andriacchi TP, Rosenberg AG (1996) Functional analysis of cemented medial unicompartmental knee arthroplasty. J Arthroplasty 11(5):553–559
17. Banks SA, Hodge WA (1996) Accurate measurement of three-dimensional knee replacement kinematics using single-plane fluoroscopy. IEEE Trans Biomed Eng 43(6):638–649
18. Tupling S, Pierrynowski M (1987) Use of Cardan angles to locate rigid bodies in three-dimensional space. Med Biol Eng Comput 25(5):527–532
19. Scott RD, Cobb AG, McQueary FG, Thornhill TS (1991) Unicompartmental knee arthroplasty. Eight- to 12-year follow-up evaluation with survivorship analysis. Clin Orthop Relat Res (271):96–100
20. Cloutier JM, Sabouret P, Deghrar A (1999) Total knee arthroplasty with retention of both cruciate ligaments. A nine to eleven-year follow-up study. J Bone Joint Surg 81-A(5):697–702
21. Stiehl JB, Komistek RD, Cloutier JM, Dennis DA (2000) The cruciate ligaments in total knee arthroplasty: a kinematic analysis of 2 total knee arthroplasties. J Arthroplasty 15(5):545–550
22. Iwaki H, Pinskerova V, Freeman MAR (2000) Tibiofemoral movement 1: the shapes and relative movements of the femur and tibia in the unloaded cadaver knee. J Bone Joint Surg 82-B:1189–1195
23. Hill PF, Vedi V, Williams A, Iwaki H, Pinskerova V, Freeman MAR (2000) Tibiofemoral movement 2: the loaded and unloaded living knee studied by MRI. J Bone Joint Surg 82-B:1196–1198
24. Komistek RD, Allain J, Anderson DT, Dennis DA, Goutallier D (2002) In vivo kinematics for subjects with and without an anterior cruciate ligament. Clin Orthop Relat Res (404):315–325
25. Insall JN, Dorr LD, Scott RD, Scott WN (1989) Rationale of the Knee Society clinical rating system. Clin Orthop Relat Res (248):13–14

26. Goodfellow JW, O'Connor J (1986) Clinical results of the Oxford knee. Surface arthroplasty of the tibiofemoral joint with a meniscal bearing prosthesis. Clin Orthop Relat Res (205):21–42

27. Blankevoort L, Huiskes R, de Lange A (1988) The envelope of passive knee joint motion. J Biomech 21(9):705–720

28. Banks SA, Markovich GD, Hodge WA (1997) The mechanics of knee replacements during gait. In vivo fluoroscopic analysis of two designs. Am J Knee Surg 10(4):261–267

29. Banks SA, Hodge WA (2004) 2003 Hap Paul Award Paper of the International Society for Technology in Arthroplasty: design and activity dependence of kinematics in fixed and mobile bearing knee arthroplasties. J Arthroplasty 19(7):809–816

MIS Patellofemoral Arthroplasty

Jess H. Lonner

The prevalence of isolated patellofemoral arthritis is high, occurring in as many as 11% of men and 24% of women older than the age of 55 years with symptomatic osteoarthritis of the knee in one study [1]. Symptomatic patellofemoral chondromalacia occurs with even greater frequency and is a very common reason for presentation for orthopedic evaluation, particularly in women between the ages of 30 and 50 years. This gender predilection is undoubtedly related to the often subtle patellar malalignment and dysplasia that is common in women. The patellofemoral cartilage is also at risk for direct traumatic injury, considering its vulnerable location in the body.

Patellofemoral arthroplasty is an attractive option for the treatment of debilitating isolated patellofemoral arthritis and diffuse grade IV patellofemoral chondromalacia. The traditional surgical alternatives, long recognized for their short-comings, are losing ground to this increasingly more popular treatment method. The pain relief resulting from patellofemoral arthroplasty is superior to other patellofemoral-specific treatment strategies, like patellectomy and tibial tubercle-unloading procedures. Additionally, enthusiasm for patellofemoral arthroplasty continues to increase as newer designs with improved features emerge, surgical indications are refined, and techniques and instrumentation improve. Furthermore, revision to total knee arthroplasty is not compromised after patellofemoral arthroplasty, making it a reasonable intermediate procedure in young and middle-aged patients with isolated patellofemoral arthritis [2].

Selecting an implant of sound design is important to optimize the ultimate results, but surgical technique, namely accurate implantation of the components and balancing the soft tissues, is paramount. The success of minimally invasive approaches to total and unicompartmental arthroplasty is creating a natural intrigue with their potential application to patellofemoral arthroplasty. It is important, however, since this is a newer treatment alternative for most, to first familiarize oneself with the nuances of the procedure through a more extensile approach, and then reduce the incision length and arthrotomy more gradually. Until recently, designs and implant systems either required completely free-handed techniques, or instruments were so large and bulky that extensile incisions and arthrotomies were necessary (Fig. 13.1). Now, particularly because of refinements in instrumentation, instrumented minimally invasive surgery (MIS) will soon be possible in patellofemoral arthroplasty.

This chapter discusses the role of patellofemoral arthroplasty for isolated patellofemoral arthritis, describes a free-handed, uninstrumented MIS surgical technique, and reviews the results of the procedure (independent of surgical approach).

J.H. Lonner (✉)
Knee Replacement Surgery, Orthopaedic Research,
Booth Bartolozzi Balderston Orthopaedics,
Pennsylvania Hospital, Philadelphia, PA, USA
e-mail: lonnerj@pahosp.com

G.R. Scuderi and A.J. Tria (eds.), *Minimally Invasive Surgery in Orthopedics: Knee Handbook*,
DOI 10.1007/978-1-4614-0679-2_13, © Springer Science+Business Media, LLC 2012

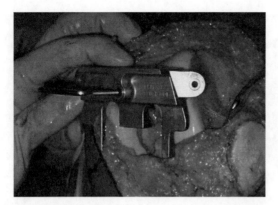

Fig. 13.1 Intraoperative photograph showing large cutting block that precludes MIS surgery

Indications and Contraindications

Patellofemoral arthroplasty may be considered in the treatment algorithm for patients with localized patellofemoral osteoarthrosis, posttraumatic arthrosis, or grade IV bipolar (involving both the patella and the trochlea) or unipolar (involving either the patella or the trochlea) chondromalacia. Oftentimes, patients will have had arthroscopic procedures and these do not preclude the opportunity for patellofemoral arthroplasty. Microfracture, autologous osteochondral transplantation plug(s), and autologous chondrocyte implantation, generally less effective in the patellofemoral compartment than in the weight bearing surfaces of the femoral condyles, are not uncommon prior to patellofemoral arthroplasty and if unsuccessful can easily be converted to patellofemoral arthroplasty.

Patellofemoral arthroplasty is appropriate for patellofemoral arthritis in the presence of dysplasia; it should be avoided in patients with considerable patellar maltracking or malalignment, unless these conditions are corrected preoperatively. Slight patellar tilt or trochlear dysplasia are not contraindications for this procedure; in such cases, a lateral retinacular release may be necessary at the time of arthroplasty [3–5]. Excessive Q angles should be corrected with tibial tubercle realignment before or simultaneous with patellofemoral arthroplasty. The procedure should not be performed in patients with inflammatory arthritis or chondrocalcinosis involving the menisci or tibiofemoral chondral surfaces, nor should it be offered to patients with diffuse pain [3–5]. Tibiofemoral arthrosis or diffuse grade III or IV chondromalacia are contraindications to patellofemoral arthroplasty, although recent work suggests a role for concomitant patellofemoral arthroplasty and biological condylar resurfacing when there is focal grade IV chondromalacia on the weight-bearing condylar surfaces noted in addition to the patellofemoral wear [6].

Patellofemoral arthroplasty is most effective in patients younger than 55 years with isolated anterior compartment arthrosis [3–5], and less predictable in elderly patients, who may be better off undergoing total knee arthroplasty.

Clinical Evaluation

History and Physical Examination

Taking a detailed history and performing a thorough physical examination of the patient under consideration for patellofemoral arthroplasty are necessary to corroborate that the pain is, in fact, localized to the anterior compartment of the knee, and that it emanates from the patellofemoral chondral surfaces and not from soft tissues (such as the patellar or quadriceps tendons or pes anserinus bursa) or other remote sites, such as the lumbar spine or ipsilateral hip.

The history should include questions about whether there was prior trauma to the knee and its mechanism, patellar dislocation, or other patellofemoral "problems." A history of recurrent atraumatic patellar dislocations may suggest considerable malalignment. Pain should characteristically be directly retropatellar, or just lateral or medial to the patella, and is often exacerbated by activities that load the patellofemoral compartment, such as stair climbing and descent, ambulating on hills, standing from a seated position, sitting with the knee flexed, and squatting. Medial or lateral joint line pain is not typical in truly isolated patellofemoral arthritis. A description of anterior crepitus is common.

The physical examination will often note pain on patella inhibition and compression, patellofemoral crepitus, and retropatellar knee pain with active and passive flexion. The presence of medial or lateral tibiofemoral joint line tenderness is concerning for the possibility of more diffuse chondral disease (even in the presence of relatively normal radiographs) and may be a contraindication to patellofemoral arthroplasty. Patellar tracking and the Q angle must be assessed, since maltracking and malalignment can compromise the outcomes after patellofemoral arthroplasty.

Imaging Studies

Standing anteroposterior and midflexion posteroanterior radiographs are critical to identify tibiofemoral arthritis. Supine coronal radiographs should be avoided because they may underestimate the presence or extent of tibiofemoral disease. Mild squaring-off of the femoral condyles and even small marginal osteophytes are not contraindications for patellofemoral arthroplasty if the patient has no tibiofemoral pain with activities and on physical exam, and if there is less than grade III chondral degeneration noted during arthroscopy or arthrotomy. Lateral X-ray results occasionally demonstrate patellofemoral osteophytes, but, particularly in younger patients, there may be minimal radiographic joint space narrowing and osteophytes; the lateral X-ray results can show whether there is patella alta or baja. Axial radiographs will demonstrate the position of the patella within the trochlear groove and the extent of arthritis, but, again, the radiographs may underestimate the extent of patellofemoral cartilage damage. Often subchondral sclerosis and facet "flattening" may be the only radiographic clues (Fig. 13.2a–c). Computed tomographic (CT) scan and magnetic resonance imaging (MRI) are not necessary for evaluating patellofemoral arthrosis, although they can be useful for evaluating patellar instability. Photographs from prior arthroscopic treatment will provide valuable information regarding the extent of anterior compartment arthrosis and the status of the tibiofemoral articular cartilage and menisci.

Surgical Technique

Like all procedures, first developing a comfort level and proficiency with a procedure and instrumentation through a more extensile arthrotomy is absolutely paramount before transitioning to minimally invasive techniques. Patellofemoral arthroplasty is unforgiving; errors in alignment and soft tissue balancing can be deleterious to the outcomes. To be clear, no surgeon should struggle with a minimally invasive approach at the expense of ensuring that the critical tenets of patellofemoral arthroplasty are fulfilled – namely, component alignment, soft tissue balance, and implant fixation. Additionally, even at present, instrumentation for patellofemoral arthroplasty has not been MIS compatible. Cutting blocks, when available, are bulky and cannot be used through less invasive arthrotomies (Fig. 13.1). Free-hand techniques, however, are more amenable to MIS approaches, but carry a risk of inaccuracy. Newer designs and instrumentation will be intended to be MIS compatible (Zimmer, Warsaw, IN).

Considering the need for exposure and preparation of the anterior surface of the femur and retropatellar surface, a small or moderate incision in the quadriceps tendon or muscle is often prudent, even advisable, particularly initially in one's early clinical experience with this procedure. As one's comfort level expands and proficiency with this procedure improves, and as newer instrumentation becomes available, a mini-subvastus approach can be utilized (Figs. 13.3a, b). The natural evolution in terms of surgical arthrotomy for patellofemoral arthrotomy should involve a standard medial parapatellar arthrotomy, followed by a standard midvastus or subvastus approach, and thereafter, mini arthrotomies can be pursued. I commonly use the gamut of MIS arthrotomies, including a mini-parapatellar limited quadriceps incision, mini-midvastus, or mini-subvastus, depending on several features, such as the presence of patellar tilt or subluxation (in those cases I try to use the mini-subvastus or mini-midvastus approach to optimize patellar tracking), the level of insertion of the vastus medialis obliquus on the patella

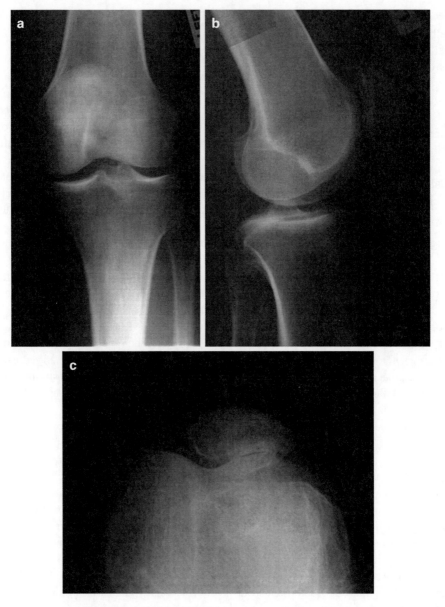

Fig. 13.2 (a–c) Weight-bearing anteroposterior, lateral, and axial radiographs demonstrating advanced patellofemoral arthrosis with sparing of the tibiofemoral compartments

(with distal insertions, I prefer a mini-parapatellar quadriceps incision or mini-midvastus incision), and the bulk and mass of the quadriceps muscle.

At its most conservative, the skin incision will extend from the medial aspect of the proximal edge of the patella (in flexion) to the joint line, just medial and proximal to the tibial tubercle (Fig. 13.4). As with all MIS approaches to the knee, the incision should be lengthened liberally if the skin edges become compromised or if there is unnecessary technical difficulty arising from the small incision or arthrotomy. During arthrotomy, it is essential to avoid cutting normal articular cartilage or the menisci. Before proceeding with patellofemoral arthroplasty, carefully inspect the entire joint to make sure the

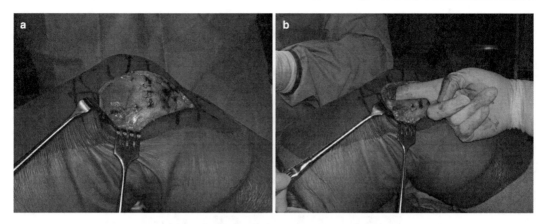

Fig. 13.3 (**a**, **b**) Defining the inferior border of the vastus medialis for a mini-subvastus approach

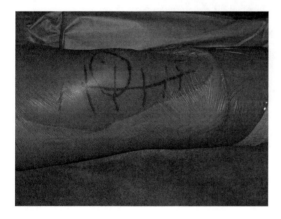

Fig. 13.4 Typical skin incision for MIS approach to patellofemoral arthroplasty

tibiofemoral compartments are free of gross cartilage degeneration.

With MIS approaches to patellofemoral arthroplasty, most of the procedure is performed with the knee either in full extension (patellar preparation), or alternating between 0 and 60° of flexion for trochlear preparation, depending on whether the anterior or posterior part of the trochlea is being prepared, respectively. My preference is to resect the articular surface of the patella before preparing the trochlea to help develop the anterior space of the knee and allow better exposure of the trochlea. This is generally done with the patella subluxed laterally and everted to 90° (Fig. 13.5a–c). The objective of patella resurfacing is to restore the original patella thickness and

medialize the component. The exposed cut surface of the lateral patella that is not covered by the patellar prosthesis should be beveled or removed to reduce the potentially painful articulation on the trochlear prosthesis in extension and mid-flexion, and on the lateral femoral condyle in deeper flexion (Fig. 13.6). It is important to avoid crushing the cut surface of the patella with the lateral retractor during trochlear preparation.

The trochlear component should be externally rotated parallel to the epicondylar axis to enhance patellar tracking; [4, 5] however, when using MIS approaches, palpation of the epicondyles is very difficult, if not impossible. Using a line perpendicular to the anteroposterior axis (which is a line drawn from the nadir of the trochlear sulcus anteriorly to the apex of the intercondylar notch posteriorly) is an accurate surrogate and my guide for component rotation in all cases unless there is profound trochlear dysplasia (Fig. 13.7). A cut is made flush with the anterior surface of the femoral cortex, avoiding notching (Figs. 13.8 and 13.9). The trochlear component should maximize coverage of the trochlea, without extending beyond the medial-lateral femoral margins anteriorly, encroaching on the weight-bearing surfaces of the tibiofemoral articulations, or overhanging into the intercondylar notch. Osteophytes bordering the intercondylar notch should be removed so that they do not impinge on the resurfaced patella or the tibia. The trochlear component edges should be flush with or recessed approximately

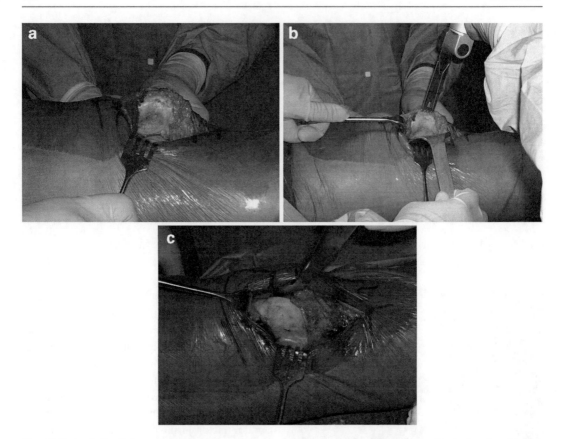

Fig. 13.5 (**a–c**) Patella preparation is performed with knee fully extended, and patella held vertically for resection. After patella preparation, exposure of the anterior femur is easier with the patella effectively reduced in size and subluxed laterally

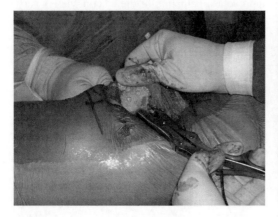

Fig. 13.6 The uncapped lateral edge of the patella is removed to prevent bony impingement

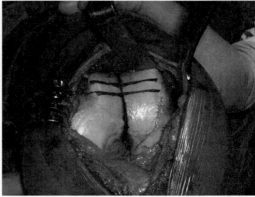

Fig. 13.7 It is the anteroposterior axis and lines perpendicular to it are marked

1 mm from the adjacent articular cartilage at the transition with the femoral condyles (Figs. 13.10 and 13.11).

Assessment of patellar tracking is performed with the trial components in place, paying particular attention to identify patellar tilt, subluxation,

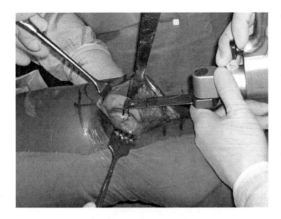

Fig. 13.8 Free-hand resection of the anterior femur, perpendicular to the anteroposterior axis, performed with the knee in approximately 30° of flexion

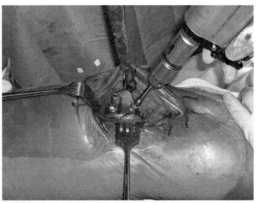

Fig. 13.11 Edges of the template are flush with the transition with the femoral condyles

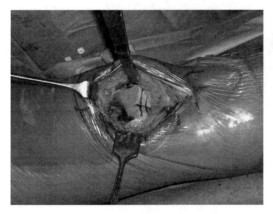

Fig. 13.9 Trochlear resection flush with the anterior surface of the femur

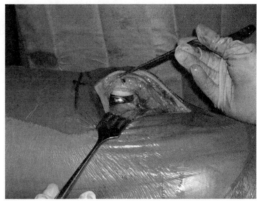

Fig. 13.12 Patellar tracking is assessed

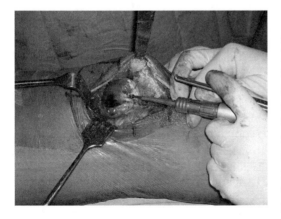

Fig. 13.10 Free-hand preparation of the distal bed for the trochlear component

or catching of the components (Fig. 13.12). Patellar tilt and mild subluxation usually can be addressed successfully by performing a lateral retinacular release, unless there is considerable extensor mechanism malalignment, which needs to be addressed with either tibial tubercle realignment (if the Q angle is excessive) or a proximal realignment. In the absence of a high Q angle, patellar maltracking with the trials in place is concerning for the possibility of component malposition. The components can then be cemented into place, removing extruded cement while it cures (Fig. 13.13a–c).

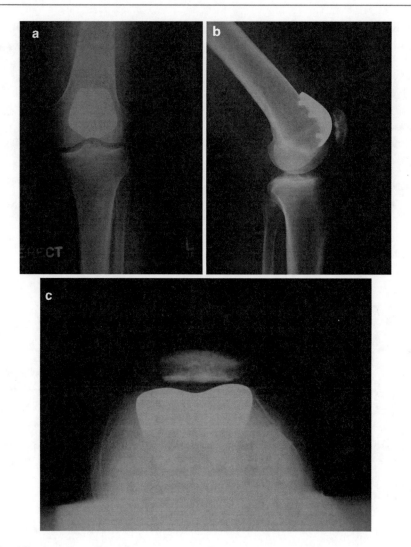

Fig. 13.13 (a–c) Postoperative radiographs

Postoperative Management

Various strategies for preemptive analgesia can be employed and these are outlined elsewhere in this book. The postoperative care is similar to that after total knee arthroplasty. A continuous passive motion machine is started immediately after surgery and used for the duration of hospitalization (average, 2 or 3 days); however, while this may accelerate early return of flexion, it is not as critical as active patient participation in flexion exercises. Isometrics and range of motion exercises are started immediately. Immediate full weight bearing is permitted, initially with the support of crutches and then a cane until there is adequate recovery of quadriceps strength. Depending on the extent of preoperative quadriceps atrophy, adequate recovery of quadriceps strength can vary; in some extreme cases, it can take 6 months or longer. Thromboembolism prophylaxis is utilized for 4–6 weeks. Twenty-four hours of perioperative antibiotics is advisable, and appropriate precautions regarding antibiotic prophylaxis for dental procedures or other interventions should follow standard recommendations of the American Academy of Orthopaedic Surgeons [7].

Clinical Results

No studies have focused specifically on how the surgical approach impacts the results of patellofemoral arthroplasty. Nonetheless, drawing from the experience of MIS total knee arthroplasty (TKA) and unicondylar knee arthroplasty (UKA), we would expect that the various MIS techniques will accelerate recovery and reduce early postoperative pain compared with standard approaches in patellofemoral arthroplasty.

Most series have reported good and excellent results in roughly 85% of cases, although there have been some outliers (Table 13.1), and the reported results in some series have been confounded by the inclusion of patients who had simultaneous patellofemoral and unicompartmental tibiofemoral arthroplasty or osteotomy, without distinguishing the clinical outcomes of those with isolated patellofemoral arthroplasties [8–12].

Results of patellofemoral arthroplasty are impacted by component position and alignment, soft tissue balance, quadriceps angle and patellofemoral alignment, implant design, indications for surgery, and presence and extent of tibiofemoral chondromalacia. Patellar instability, resulting from soft tissue imbalance, component malposition, or extensor mechanism malalignment, is the major source of short- and mid-term failure in patellofemoral arthroplasty, and a prominent source of residual anterior knee pain [5, 9, 13–16]. Improved designs have substantially reduced the incidence of patellofemoral complications [5]. In the reported series, less than 1% of patellofemoral arthroplasties have failed because of loosening or wear of the implants, although follow-up in most series has averaged less than 7 years [5, 9, 13–18].

One series has highlighted how the trochlear shape can impact the incidence of patellofemoral-related problems [5]. Thirty consecutive patellofemoral arthroplasties using one implant were compared with 25 consecutive patellofemoral arthroplasties using another implant. Patients in each group had similar demographic characteristics and preoperative range of motion and knee scores. Overall, satisfactory results were noted in 84% of patellofemoral arthroplasties, but the incidence of patellofemoral dysfunction, including subluxation, catching, and substantial pain was 17% with one prosthesis and less than 4% with the other [5].

The design characteristics of the trochlear component geometry that impact patellofemoral mechanics and tracking include the sagittal radius of curvature, the proximal extension of the anterior flange, the width of the anterior surface of the implant, and the degree of constraint. Trochlear implants with an obtuse radius of curvature commonly end up malpositioned, with the implant flexed and offset proximally from the anterior surface of the femoral cortex or extending off the bone in the intercondylar region of the knee. The former problem can often result in patellar snapping, clunking, and maltracking in the initial 30° of flexion as the distal edge of the patellar implant transitions over the proximal edge of the trochlear implant; the latter causes similar mechanical symptoms as the knee is extended from deep flexion, if the proximal edge of the patellar component impinges on the prominent distal edge of the trochlear component, or it can cause impingement on the tibia or anterior cruciate ligament (ACL) in extension. Trochlear components with a radius of curvature that mates better with most distal femora have a lesser tendency to have these problems. Broader anterior surfaces allow more freedom for patellar excursion and tracking than narrow implants. Implants with limited proximal extension on the anterior femur are susceptible to patellar prosthesis snapping and catching at the point of transition from the anterior femoral surface in full extension onto the trochlear prosthesis at approximately 10–30° of flexion; again, this is hastened if the trochlear component is flexed or offset anteriorly. This is less likely with a trochlear prosthesis that extends further proximally because the patellar component articulates entirely with the trochlear component in extension.

Table 13.1 Clinical results of MIS patellofemoral arthroplasty

Series	Implant	Number of PFAs	Age (years)	Diagnosis	Duration of follow-up	Percentage of good/excellent results (%)
Blazina [13]	Richards types I and II	57	39 (range, 19–81)	NA	2 years (range, 8–42 months)	NA
Arciero [8]	Richards type II (14); CFS-Wright (11)	25	62 (range, 33–86)	OA (25); malalignment or instability (14)	5.3 years (range, 3–9 years)	85
Cartier [9]	Richards types II and III	72	65 (range, 23–89)	Dysplasia/grade IV chondromalacia (29); PTA (3); chondrocalcinosis (5)	4 years (range, 2–12 years)	85
Argenson [10]	Autocentric	66	57 (range, 19–82)	Dysplasia or dislocation (22); PTA (20); OA (24)	5.5 years (range, 2–10 years)	84
Krajca [20]	Richards types I and II	16	64 (range, 42–84)	Primary OA (10); PTA (2); recurrent dislocation (1)	5.8 years (range, 2–18 years)	88
Tauro [15]	Lubinus	62	66 (range, 50–87)	PTA (2); primary OA (74)	7.5 years (range 5–10 years)	45
deWinter [14]	Richards type II	26	59 (range, 22–90)	Primary OA (17); malalignment (8); PTA (1)	11 years (range, 1–20 years)	76
Ackroyd [16]	Avon	306	62 (range, 34–92)	Primary OA (187); dysplasia (12); subluxation/dislocation (41); PTA (5); other (4)	NA	NA
Smith [17]	Lubinus	45	72 (range, 42–86)	Primary OA (44); PTA (1)	4 years (range, 6 months–7.5 years)	69
Kooijman [19]	Richards type II	45	50 (range, 20–77)	OA (45)	17 years (range, 15–21 years)	86
Lonner [5]	Lubinus	30	38 (range, 34–51)	Primary OA (26); PTA (4); s/p tibial tubercle realignment (10)	4 years (range, 2–6 years)	84
Lonner [5]	Avon trochlea; Nexgen patella	25	44 (range, 28–59)	Primary OA (25); s/p realignment (2)	6 months (range, 1 month–1 year)	96
Merchant [18]	LCS	15	49 (range, 30–81)	Subluxation/dislocation (12); PTA (2); osteochondritis dissecans (1)	3.75 years (range, 2.25–5.5 years)	93
Cartier [11]	Richards types II and III	59	60 (range, 36–81)	Primary OA (7); dysplasia/subluxation (41); grade IV chondromalacia (4); PTA (3); s/p realignment (13)	10 years (range, 6–16 years)	72

PFA patellofemoral arthroplasty, *NA* not applicable, *OA* osteoarthritis, *PTA* posttraumatic arthrosis, *LCS* low contact stress

The problem may be compounded by the degree of trochlear constraint (manifest by the sulcus angle) in the axial plane. An increased degree of freedom within the trochlear groove is more forgiving in extension than those implants with lower sulcus angles, and less likely to cause wear of the patellar component or dynamic tracking problems.

Several studies have reported the long-term outcomes after patellofemoral arthroplasty. Tibiofemoral degeneration is the most common reason for late "failures" of patellofemoral arthroplasties. Kooijman et al. reported that after a mean of 15.6 years (range, 10–21 years), 25% of 45 patellofemoral arthroplasties required secondary surgeries for progressive tibiofemoral arthritis, including two proximal tibial osteotomies and ten total knee arthroplasties. In other words, 75% of the implants studied were still functioning well into the second decade after implantation. Of those patellofemoral implants that were still in place, 86% were considered successful [19]. Cartier et al. performed an analysis of 59 patellofemoral arthroplasties from a cohort of 117 [11]. A large number had previous or concomitant surgeries, including tibial tubercle realignment procedures or soft tissue surgeries for patellofemoral maltracking. At a mean follow-up of 10 years (range, 6–16 years), 47 knees were pain free and 12 had moderate or severe pain, primarily from tibiofemoral arthritis, but also from lateral patellar subluxation in one knee and trochlear soft tissue impingement in two. Stair ambulation was considered normal in 91% of patients. Knee Society knee scores were excellent (77%), fair (14%), and poor (9%); Knee Society function scores were excellent (72%), fair (19%), and poor (9%). No cases of patellar or trochlear loosening were identified. Patellar snapping was observed in 2% of cases. Substantial polyethylene wear was present in one case and moderate in five. There were two drop off points on the survivorship curve: an early one, at 3 years, related to inappropriate indications for the surgery, and another in the 9th and 10th years, corresponding to the development of symptomatic tibiofemoral osteoarthritis. The authors reported a survivorship of 75% at 11 years [11].

In a series by Argenson et al., the best results were achieved after patellofemoral arthroplasty performed for posttraumatic arthritis (resulting from patella fracture) or patellar subluxation and dysplasia, and the least favorable in those with primary degenerative arthritis. The development of tibiofemoral arthritis was the most frequent cause of failure [10, 12]. In 66 patellofemoral arthroplasties in patients with a mean age of 57 years (range, 21–82 years) and with a mean follow-up of 16.2 years (range, 12–20 years), there were 14 concomitant procedures, including nine tibiofemoral osteotomies and five distal patellar realignments. While most patients had substantial and sustained pain relief, 25% were revised to TKA for tibiofemoral arthritis (at a mean of 7.3 years after patellofemoral arthroplasty), 14% for aseptic trochlear component loosening (at a mean of 4.5 years after patellofemoral arthroplasty; 38% of which were uncemented designs), and 5% for infection. In those who retained their patellofemoral arthroplasties at most recent follow-up, Knee Society knee and function scores improved from 53 (range, 43–70) to 79 (range, 60–100), and 41 (range, 10–80) to 81 (range, 40–100), respectively. The cumulative 16-year survivorship was 58%, but the authors continue to advocate for the procedure as an intermediate stage before TKA in the absence of tibiofemoral arthritis or coronal plane malalignment [12].

Summary

Patellofemoral arthroplasty can be an effective treatment for patellofemoral arthritis resulting from primary osteoarthrosis, dysplasia, or posttraumatic arthrosis in young and middle-aged patients who have normal patellofemoral alignment without considerable maltracking or subluxation. The results of patellofemoral arthroplasty can be impacted by the design features of the trochlear component, the presence of uncorrectable patellar instability or malalignment, implant malposition (potentially hastened by particular designs), and tibiofemoral chondromalacia or arthrosis. Evolving designs can reduce considerably the incidence of patellofemoral dysfunction, leaving progressive tibiofemoral arthritis as the primary potential failure mechanisms of patellofemoral arthroplasty. If the early patellofemoral failures are excluded, the short-term failure rate is reduced.

As with all knee procedures, MIS techniques can be applied to patellofemoral arthroplasty, but only after the procedure has been performed effectively and accurately through more extensile approaches. MIS may be particularly effective in this patient cohort, which often has significant preoperative quadriceps atrophy associated with the advanced patellofemoral arthritis, because minimizing trauma to the extensor mechanism during surgery may reduce the problem of iatrogenic postoperative quadriceps atrophy. The surgical approach should not negatively impact the outcome of patellofemoral arthroplasty because of errors in implantation or fixation, but instead should facilitate the experience, accelerate the recovery, and not impact the long-term outcomes. That is what MIS, done well, can provide.

References

1. McAlindon RE, Snow S, Cooper C, Dieppe PA. Radiographic patterns of osteoarthritis of the knee joint in the community: The importance of the patellofemoral joint. Ann Rheum Dis 51:844–849, 1992
2. Lonner JH, Jasko JG, Booth RE. Revision of a failed patellofemoral arthroplasty to a total knee arthroplasty. J Bone Joint Surg (Am) 88:2337–2342, 2006
3. Lonner JH. Patellofemoral arthroplasty. Semin Arthroplasty 11:234–240, 2000
4. Lonner JH. Patellofemoral arthroplasty. Tech Knee Surg 2:144–152, 2003
5. Lonner JH. Patellofemoral arthroplasty: pros, cons, design considerations. Clin Orthop Relat Res (428): 158–165, 2004
6. Lonner JH, Mehta S, Jasko JG. Ipsilateral patellofemoral arthroplasty and femoral condylar osteochondral autograft. J Arthroplasty (in press)
7. Hanssen AD, Osmon DR, Nelson CL. Prevention of deep periprosthetic joint infection. J Bone Joint Surg 78A:458–471, 1996
8. Arciero R, Toomey H: Patellofemoral arthroplasty. A three to nine year follow-up study. Clin Orthop Relat Res (236):60–71, 1988
9. Cartier P, Sanouiller JL, Grelsamer R. Patellofemoral arthroplasty. J Arthroplasty 5:49–55, 1990
10. Argenson JN, Guillaume JM, Aubaniac JM. Is there a place for patellofemoral arthroplasty? Clin Orthop Relat Res (321):162–167, 1995
11. Cartier P, Sanouiller JL, Khefacha A. Long-term results with the first patellofemoral prosthesis. Clin Orthop Relat Res (436):4754, 2005
12. Argenson JN, Flecher X, Parratte S, Aubaniac JM. Patellofemoral arthroplasty: an update. Clin Orthop Relat Res (440):50–53, 2005
13. Blazina ME, Fox JM, Del Pizzo W, Broukhim B, Ivey FM. Patellofemoral replacement. Clin Orthop Relat Res (144):98–102, 1979
14. deWinter WE, Feith R, van Loon CJ. The Richards type II patellofemoral arthroplasty: 26 cases followed for 1–20 years. Acta Orthop Scand 72: 487–490, 2001
15. Tauro B, Ackroyd CE, Newman JH, Shah NA. The Lubinus patellofemoral arthroplasty. A five to ten year prospective study. J Bone Joint Surg 83B: 696–701, 2001
16. Ackroyd CE, Newman JH, Webb JM, Eldridge JDJ. The Avon patellofemoral arthroplasty. Two to five year results. *Proceedings of the American Academy of Orthopaedic Surgeons.* New Orleans, LA, February 2003
17. Smith AM, Peckett WRC, Butler-Manuel PA, Venu KM, d'Arey JC. Treatment of patellofemoral arthritis using the Lubinus patellofemoral arthroplasty. A retrospective review. Knee 9:27–30, 2002
18. Merchant AC. Early results with a total patellofemoral joint replacement arthroplasty prosthesis. J Arthroplasty 19:829–836, 2004
19. Kooijman HJ, Driessen APPM, van Horn JR. Long-term results of patellofemoral arthroplasty. J Bone Joint Surg 85-B:836–840, 2003
20. Krajca-Radcliffe JB, Coker TP. Patellofemoral arthroplasty. A 2 to 18 year follow up study. Clin Orthop Relat Res 330:143–151, 1996

Round Table Discussion of MIS Total Knee Arthroplasty

14

Giles R. Scuderi, Mark W. Pagnano, Steven B. Haas, Richard A. Berger, Alfred J. Tria Jr., and Peter Bonutti

Giles R. Scuderi: Minimally invasive surgery (MIS) total knee arthroplasty (TKA) has become a popular surgical technique. Surgeons are performing the procedure through smaller skin incisions and limited arthrotomies. Yet this is not a technique for all patients and all surgeons. I have gathered a

G.R. Scuderi (✉)
Insall Scott Kelly Institute for Orthopaedics
and Sports Medicine, New York, NY, USA
e-mail: gscuderi@iskinstitute.com

North Shore-LIJ Health System, Great Neck, NY, USA

Albert Einstein College of Medicine, New York,
NY, USA

M.W. Pagnano
Department of Orthopaedic Surgery, Mayo Clinic
College of Medicine, Mayo Clinic, Rochester, MN, USA

S.B. Haas
Department of Orthopedic Surgery,
Hospital for Special Surgery, New York, NY, USA

Weill Medical College of Cornell University, New York,
NY, USA

R.A. Berger
Department of Orthopaedic Surgery, Rush-
Presbyterian-St. Luke's Medical Center, Chicago,
IL, USA

A.J. Tria Jr.
Institute for Advanced Orthopaedic Study, The
Orthopaedic Center of New Jersey, Somerset, NJ, USA

Department of Orthopedic Surgery, Robert Wood
Johnson Medical School, Piscataway, NJ, USA

P. Bonutti
Bonutti Clinic, Effingham, IL, USA

Department of Orthopaedics, University of Arkansas,
Little Rock, AR, USA

group of experts who will share their experiences. This panel includes Mark Pagnano, Steven Haas, Richard Berger, Alfred Tria, and Peter Bonutti. Let us start this discussion with patient selection. My own experience has shown that MIS total knee arthroplasty is more applicable to a thin female patient with minimal deformity and good preoperative range of motion. Mark, is there a way of determining who is an ideal candidate for a minimally invasive total knee?

Mark Pagnano: For me, the easiest patient is the elderly female patient who is slightly overweight and has moderate angular deformity with a reasonable range of motion. The patient who is somewhat overweight has some of that adipose tissue distributed within the muscle and that makes the muscle and soft tissue easier to mobilize during surgery. A moderate angular deformity allows me to do some ligamentous release early in the case and that facilitates both visualization and the placement of retractors under direct vision to protect the collateral ligaments and the posterior neurovascular structures. A small flexion contracture is of no concern but I like to see at least 100° of flexion. Finally, the ideal patient will require tibial and femoral implant sizes that are in the small to medium size range; the largest implants often have a dimension that approaches the skin incision size and those are difficult to maneuver into place gracefully.

Giles R. Scuderi: With these variables in mind, Steve, which patients are better served with a more traditional approach?

Steve Haas: It is generally much easier to perform MIS total knee arthroplasty in female patients. Large muscular men are the most difficult. Men that are heavier than 210–220 lb will receive a larger arthrotomy extending into the quadriceps and a proportionally larger incision. It is, however, not necessary to evert the patella in these patients. Patients with severe deformities, particularly flexion contractures greater than 20–25°, require a standard medial parapatellar arthrotomy. Additionally stiff patients with flexion less than 80° are not good candidates for MIS TKA.

Giles R. Scuderi: Rich, Mark, and Steve have nicely outlined the patient factors, but what about the surgeon? What are your recommendations for the surgeons beginning to learn this technique?

Rich Berger: Fortunately, minimally invasive total knee arthroplasty is perfectly situated for a stepwise approach to getting started. I recommend first becoming accustomed to your minimally invasive instruments using whichever approach you are most familiar with – for most, this will be a medial parapatellar approach. Then as you become facile with the instruments, begin making a smaller arthrotomy without everting the patella. If you experience difficulty during a case, simply extend the arthrotomy. With more experience, further reduce the arthrotomy, eventually using a capsular-only incision (such as Fred will address) or explore other approaches such as a mini-midvastus or mini-subvastus, both of which give you more exposure than the capsular-only incision. However, both the mini-midvastus and mini-subvastus will self-extend as you stress the tissues; thus, becoming closer to standard midvastus or standard subvastus. While this self-extension aids exposure, it is difficult to control and will hinder the patient's recovery. I believe that the limited medial parapatellar and the capsular only incision does not self-extend; you control exactly how much exposure you have by the length of the capsular incision.

Giles R. Scuderi: Rich, I agree with you, that is why I prefer a limited medial parapatellar arthrotomy that can be lengthened as I need to gain exposure. It is an approach with which I have a great deal of experience and feel the most comfortable and believe can be used in the vast major-

ity of case. I also use instruments that are similar to my traditional instruments. The only difference is that they are reduced in size to fit within the limited arthrotomy. Now, Fred, in contrast, you are doing your cases through a quadriceps-sparing approach. How difficult is that? Did you not have to change the way you do the knee?

Fred Tria: Initially, we had to change the surgical technique quite a bit to accommodate the limited incision for the quadriceps-sparing approach. We resected the patellar surface first to increase the overall space in the knee. The distal femoral cut was made from the medial side, as was the proximal tibial resection. The finishing blocks for the femur were cut down and the alignment guides for the block were unique. We used grasping hooks on the posterior aspect of the tibial finishing plates and modified the tibial tray by decreasing the length of the intramedullary stem. Our accuracy was not as good as the standard arthrotomy and we looked for a way to simplify the technique. Now, we use instruments that are more standard that allow the surgeon to cut from anterior to posterior with improved methods for exposure of the bone. We hope that these efforts in combination with navigation will show improvement in the overall accuracy.

Giles R. Scuderi: But, Fred, you know it is a struggle to work through such a very limited arthrotomy and I am always concerned that I may not be seeing enough of the joint to accurately cut the femur and tibia and then get the implant into the joint. Yet, I do applaud your efforts to preserve the integrity of the extensor mechanism. Steve, you use the midvastus approach, do you think it has an advantage over the quadriceps-sparing technique?

Steve Haas: I believe it is easier to gain adequate exposure to the knee with a mini-midvastus approach compared with a "quad-sparing" technique. There is much better access to the front of the femur, and it is much easier to expose the tibia for tibial component insertion. The "quad-sparing" technique also stretches the vastus medialis oblique (VMO) to a much greater extent than the mini-midvastus approach. Clinical results have been equal for the two approaches and I believe the learning curve for the mini-midvastus approach is shorter.

Giles R. Scuderi: Steve, I must say, when I have used the midvastus approach, the fascia would split proximally until the vastus medialis is released. Have you seen this and do you think it really matters?

Steve Haas: While the VMO can spread further in a midvastus approach, our studies indicate that there is less spreading with the "mini" midvastus approach than the standard midvastus approach. Even with a standard midvastus approach with greater splitting, long-term studies have shown no persistent electromyogram (EMG) changes from this muscle splitting. Generally, the amount splitting with the mini-midvastus approach is less than 2–3 cm, and we have not seen any splits greater than 4 cm.

Giles R. Scuderi: Peter, You also use a midvastus approach, do you have anything to add?

Peter Bonutti: I have used numerous approaches, the mini-midvastus, mini-subvastus, and direct lateral approach. We have performed prospective randomized studies using isokinetic analysis and have found that the mini-midvastus approach seems to have less pain postoperatively, but via isokinetic analysis, the subvastus approach appears to have faster quadriceps recovery. Currently, we have evolved from a mini-midvastus and now use a modified mini-subvastus approach and are able to do this universally in all patients. Using the mini-subvastus approach, it is more difficult to obtain exposure to the femur, but use of this approach may allow slightly faster recovery of the quadriceps mechanism.

Giles R. Scuderi: Peter, I agree and think those are great comments. But I do need to ask Mark, with the subvastus approach, you suggest that this is also a quadriceps-sparing approach, do you think it is easier then the midvastus approach? I have found that if the vastus medialis is bulky it is difficult to laterally sublux the patella.

Mark Pagnano: The key to visualization with the MIS subvastus approach is to understand that the inferior fibers of the vastus medialis insert at a 50° angle relative to the long axis of the femur and that the tendon of the vastus medialis extends all the way to the mid-pole of the patella. One must preserve that triangular extension of tendon

down to the mid-pole because that is where your retractor will rest when you translate the patella into the lateral gutter. By preserving that triangular portion of tendon above the mid-pole you gain two benefits: first the retractor will always rest against a robust edge of tendon so the vastus medialis itself does not become cut, split, or macerated and, second, you gain a geometric advantage so that as you retract the patella laterally the vastus medialis drapes over the anterior femur and not over the distal femur. When surgeons have difficulty translating the patella laterally it is usually because the approach into the subvastus space has been made too horizontally. A horizontal capsular incision often results in a portion of the medial patellofemoral ligament remaining intact and that will limit lateral translation of the patella. Instead, the capsular incision into the subvastus interval should parallel the inferior fibers of the vastus medialis and that means extending it at a 50° angle from inferior to superior starting at the mid-pole of the patella.

Giles R. Scuderi: Rich, it seems as I listen to my colleagues, the real issue is whether the extensor mechanism is partially released or not and the whether or not the patella is laterally subluxed. Does it really matter and is there a significant difference in the clinical outcome?

Rich Berger: Ideally, there should be little difference in the approaches if all approaches used very small instruments, did not evert the patella under tension, did not stress the surrounding tissues, and did not dislocate the knee. Any approach, done mostly in extension with minimal retraction of the extensor mechanism, should similarly benefit our patients. Unfortunately, most instruments are still too large and are used in flexion where retractors stress the extensor mechanism. In this environment, I believe that the approaches that can self-extend (midvastus and subvastus) do extend significantly under the skin. Therefore, the mini-midvastus and mini-subvastus become close to a standard midvastus and standard subvastus; these standard approaches clearly are not as beneficial to the patients as approaches that limit the detachment of the quadriceps.

I have done a significant number of cases with each of the four approaches discussed here.

I believe, the more exposure you have, the more trauma you are causing for the patient; therefore, some struggle is necessary to help your patient recover more rapidly postoperatively. From this experience, I have found that the capsularly only exposure cause the least trauma and has the best results in my hands; however, it also affords the least exposure.

Giles R. Scuderi: I would like to summarize the surgical approaches by saying that there are several techniques to perform the total knee arthroplasty, but it is important that the surgeon know his options and not compromise the clinical outcome. In choosing an approach, there must be an option for extending the exposure in order to gain full exposure. Now let's talk about specific issues and start with correction of fixed deformities. Fred, how do you manage the fixed varus deformity with a MIS quadriceps-sparing technique?

Fred Tria: The varus deformity is not difficult to correct with the quadriceps-sparing approach because the dissection is right in the operative field on the medial side of the knee. The deep medial collateral ligament is always released as part of the initial exposure and the posterior medial capsule is also visible with this early release. The insertion of the semimembranosus can be exposed by externally rotating the tibia with the knee flexed approximately 30°. The superficial medial collateral ligament can be released by using a periosteal elevator beneath the ligament and tapping the instrument distally along the medial tibial metaphysis beneath the insertion of the pes anserinus. If a complete release is necessary, the insertion of the medial collateral over the fascia of the soleus muscle can be released with a knife along the posterior medial corner of the tibia. A complete release with the quadriceps-sparing approach would rarely be necessary because we limit the indications to a knee that has no more than 10° of fixed varus deformity. The valgus deformity can be approached with the quadriceps-sparing technique but it is slightly more difficult because all of the releases are on the opposite side of the joint. We do not recommend a lateral arthrotomy approach for the quadriceps-sparing technique.

Giles R. Scuderi: I would agree. Mark, what about a fixed valgus deformity, can you correct it with the subvastus approach and, if so, how do you do it?

Mark Pagnano: The fixed valgus deformity is easily addressed with the subvastus technique. A contemporary method of dealing with the valgus deformity is the so-called pie-crusting or multiple puncture technique. The initial bone cuts are performed on the tibia and the femur and a spacer block is placed in the extension space and then in the flexion space to determine the relative symmetry between the medial and lateral sides. When the lateral side is found to be tight, we bring the leg into extension and place a laminar spreader in the extension space. In full extension, there is no substantial tension on the extensor mechanism and the subvastus approach affords an unobstructed view of the extension space. The surgeon can then palpate the lateral-sided structures including the iliotibial band, the fibular collateral ligament, the posterolateral capsule, and the popliteus tendon and decide which structure is tightest. Multiple small punctures are then made in the tightest structure with a #15 blade, using care not to plunge toward the peroneal nerve in the posterolateral corner. If release of one structure is insufficient to balance the lateral side with the medial side, then sequential multiple puncture release of the next tightest structure is carried out until a rectangular extension gap is obtained.

Giles R. Scuderi: Peter, how about ligament balancing with the suspended leg technique? Do you find it easier to correct deformities and do you have any comments about femoral component rotation?

Peter Bonutti: The suspended leg technique has a number of advantages. The procedure is performed with the knee primarily in flexion, distracted by gravity. This may enhance exposure to the distal femur. One needs to use caution on femoral rotation with the suspended leg approach as the extremity may be rotated with use of the retractors because the extremity is free to rotate. Gravity for distraction can enhance exposure and, by applying torsional stress and variably flexing and extending the joint with the surgeon in a seated position, it can enhance exposure to the joint and may assist in true ligament balancing.

Giles R. Scuderi: I think all of you have clearing reinforced the point that the surgical principles have not changed with the MIS approaches. I do find however that the placement of the components is sometimes difficult and, for that reason, I put the tibia in first, followed by the femoral component, and then the tibial polyethylene. If I am unable to sublux the tibia forward, I insert the tibial polyethylene in mid flexion, approximately 60–70°. This is easy with a front-loading tibial tray. Fred, how do you do it with the quadriceps-sparing approach?

Fred Tria: We also insert the tibial tray first and prefer the MIS type tibia with a more limited intramedullary stem. Initially, we were inserting the tray into the knee with the knee in almost full extension. Now, with more experience in the exposure, we have been able to sublux the tibia forward in approximately 80° of flexion and place the tray on the top of the cut surface. This permits more accurate tray placement and easier cement removal. The components are cemented with separately mixed batches to allow time for each step. The femur is inserted with a holder attached to it and with the knee flexed approximately 70°. The polyethylene is inserted with the knee flexed approximately 30° with the front-loading design. The patella does not have to be resurfaced but we do so in all of our cases. This is performed as the last step, with the knee in full extension, using some of the remaining cement from the femoral prosthesis.

Giles R. Scuderi: As you all are aware, I prefer a posterior stabilized implant for all my cases and find it easier to perform a minimally invasive approach with this implant design because once you release the anterior cruciate ligament (ACL) and posterior cruciate ligament (PCL), both the flexion and extension gaps open up and it is easier to manipulate the knee and insert the components and balance the knee. Rich, how about with a cruciate-retaining knee design, do you find a difference?

Rich Berger: I have used both cruciate-retaining and cruciate-substituting designs in MIS total knee approaches; I see no clear advantage of one design over the other for minimally invasive approaches. I have found that retaining the cruciate ligament makes the exposure slightly more difficult and the bone cuts slightly harder to make. However, without a femoral box and without a keel on the tibial component (a four-peg tibial design), component placement is slightly easier in a cruciate-retaining design. Conversely, in the cruciate-substituting designs, the exposure is slightly better when the PCL is released and the bone cuts are easier to make, however, as you mentioned above, final component placement is harder due to the femoral box and the tibial keel. (The advent of the mini keel tibial component and the modular tibial component has made component placement in a cruciate-substituting designs easier, but still more difficult than a cruciate-retaining design.) Since there is no clear advantage of one design over the other, I would stronger recommend that the surgeon stay with the design they are most familiar with when moving to minimally invasive total knee techniques.

Giles R. Scuderi: How about cement versus cementless fixation? Rich, aren't you doing cementless knees?

Rich Berger: Even in large standard incisions, removing all the excess cement is difficult. Retained cement, acting as a third body, is one of the most significant causes of wear in our retrieval study of well-functioning total knees. Smaller incisions make it more difficult to properly cement components and remove excess cement. Therefore, I believe that the use of cementless knees will increase in the near future, just as cementless fixation for total hips has evolved to be the major form of fixation. Personally, I do many hybrid total knees (cementless femoral fixation). I believe that as cementless fixation improves, especially with trabecular metal, that I will do more cementless femoral and tibial fixation. I am not sure if I will ever feel comfortable using cementless patella fixation.

Giles R. Scuderi: With the evolution of MIS TKA, came improved clinical pathways, especially pain management. I am now using preemptive analgesics, regional blocks, and improved postoperative pain management techniques, which, along with a team approach with rehabilitation and nursing, has improved patient satisfaction and reduced the length of stay. Mark, I know that you have a specific pain management protocol. Can you share with us your experience?

Mark Pagnano: We have found that effective postoperative pain management markedly improves patient satisfaction, decreases hospital stays, and facilitates discharge to home instead of to rehabilitation or nursing centers. The emphasis has been to use a comprehensive multimodal approach and to be preemptive. By using multiple modalities, you can often stay below the threshold for side effects and, by staying ahead of the pain, these patients end up using less opioid medication. The focus of our approach is to eliminate the use of parenteral opioid medication altogether. Preoperatively patients are given a COX-II anti-inflammatory, acetaminophen, and a sustained-release oral opioid. Intraoperatively, patients have a femoral nerve block done and an indwelling catheter is left for the first two nights after surgery. Patients also have a single shot sciatic nerve block because the femoral block alone fails to address posterior knee pain after surgery. A short-acting spinal anesthetic and intravenous sedation is used during the total knee surgery. Postoperatively patients are given medication on a schedule in an effort to stay ahead of the pain: a sustained-release oral opioid (OxyContin) is given twice daily for the first 2 days, acetaminophen is given three times daily, Celebrex is given twice daily and oxycodone is available on an as-needed basis for breakthrough pain. Patients can ambulate toe-touch weight-bearing on day 1 even with the femoral nerve catheter in place. Thus, physical therapy does not need to be delayed, but patients can not put full weight on the leg until the femoral nerve catheter has been pulled. With this protocol, the pain scores on a verbal analog scale routinely are zero to two throughout the entire 2- or 3-day hospitalization and patients are discharged on acetaminophen, the COX-II anti-inflammatory, and a short-acting oral opioid.

Giles R. Scuderi: Rich, I am fascinated that you are now able to perform MIS total knee arthroplasty as an ambulatory procedure? How do you do it?

Rich Berger: Outpatient total knee replacement is a comprehensive approach to the patient. This includes the surgery, perioperative anesthesia and pain management, preoperative patient education, and rapid rehabilitation protocols. Clearly, starting with a minimally invasive surgical technique, done without detecting or cutting into the quadriceps is imperative. I do the procedure mostly in extension, without patella eversion, with little tension on the surrounding tissues. This technique allows less perioperative anesthesia and pain medications. The combination of less soft tissue injury with less medication allows patients to ambulate with only a cane or no assistive device within a few hours after the procedure in most patients. With little pain and little functional deficients, most of my patients choose to go home the day of surgery. My perioperative pathways and pain management protocol is similar to what Mark discussed above. However, without releasing the vastus off the intramuscular septum, without dislocating the knee, and without stressing the extensor mechanism, almost all of my capsular-only incision total knee replacement patients go home the day of surgery.

Giles R. Scuderi: Peter, how about deep vein thrombosis (DVT) prophylaxis and anticoagulation with a rapid recovery protocol? What is your current practice?

Peter Bonutti: I think anticoagulation is an important issue. Many surgeons who use rapid recovery do not use postoperative anticoagulation. In our limited study, we have found a substantive difference between those patients who utilize anticoagulation (Coumadin, Lovenox, Heparin) versus those patients who use aspirin and pulsatile stockings. The patients who use aspirin and pulsatile stockings clearly recover faster and have less postoperative pain, so this may be an important adjunct factor. The faster recovery and immediate range of motion (ROM) and weightbearing may decrease the risk for DVT and this needs to be evaluated because clearly there is a substantial difference in recovery between these two groups.

Giles R. Scuderi: Well, I want to thank all of you for sharing with me your tips and pearls in performing MIS total knee arthroplasty. This has been a very insightful and enlightening discussion. While the surgical technique has drifted toward smaller incisions and limited arthrotomies, the well-established principles of total knee arthroplasty have not changed. Adequate exposure is needed to appropriately correct deformities and balance the knee, restore alignment, and secure component fixation. These principles must not be compromised in favor of a smaller incision. It also appears that it is not the surgical technique alone, but the newer clinical pathways that have influenced clinical outcomes.

Computer-Assisted Orthopedic Surgery (CAOS): Pros and Cons

15

James B. Stiehl

Computer-assisted orthopedic surgery (CAOS) has recently evolved as an important technical application that has offered substantial improvements over conventional instrumented methods. The possibility of using computers in total joint replacement surgery is not a recent discovery, as Bargar and Paul introduced the first successful robotic application for total hips in 1987 [1]. Their system was a development effort with IBM, which had identified a considerable research program to apply robotics to medicine. Perhaps the most significant discovery at the time was to refine digital software algorithms to the level of "pixel accuracy" (20–30 mm). This was required for the machining of custom total hip femoral implants that were implanted at that time. The next years of evolution occurred in Europe, where computer algorithms were advanced to allow intraoperative registration, removing the need for preoperative fiducial placement. DiGioia and Jaramaz developed the first computed tomography (CT) system that could be applied for navigation of the acetabular component [2]. Actually, this approach was a step backward because the complex robot was not needed. Imageless total knee applications were an even simpler method because preoperative images were no longer needed.

From a purely scientific point of view, the proof of these systems for increasing surgical precision and presumed benefit has been straightforward.

The literature that I will outline clearly indicates the benefit of computer-assisted techniques over conventional instrumentation. Even in imageless total hip applications with lesser accuracy, computer-assisted surgery (CAS) provides a statistical improvement over conventional techniques from most studies. In this chapter, I offer a broad overview of the current state of the art. As with minimally invasive surgery (MIS), there are a group of early advocates who may offer a more enthusiastic viewpoint. As demonstrated, I will describe my current experience and research, which would question some of the claims regarding electromagnetic applications and imageless total hip applications, for example. However, this technology is a moving target, and improvements are being developed as we speak.

Literature Review

Total Knee Arthroplasty

Numerous authors have investigated outcomes after total knee arthroplasty (TKA), finding that malalignment of greater than 3° resulted in a significantly higher potential for mechanical loosening and implant failure. Petersen and Engh investigated the radiographic results of 50 patients who underwent primary TKA with conventional methods, noting a 26% failure to achieve alignment within the optimum of 3° of varus or valgus [3]. Berend et al. investigated tibial component failure mechanisms, noting that malalignment of

J.B. Stiehl (✉)
Department of Orthopaedic Surgery,
Medical College of Wisconsin, Milwaukee, WI, USA
e-mail: jbstiehl@me.com

G.R. Scuderi and A.J. Tria (eds.), *Minimally Invasive Surgery in Orthopedics: Knee Handbook*,
DOI 10.1007/978-1-4614-0679-2_15, © Springer Science+Business Media, LLC 2012

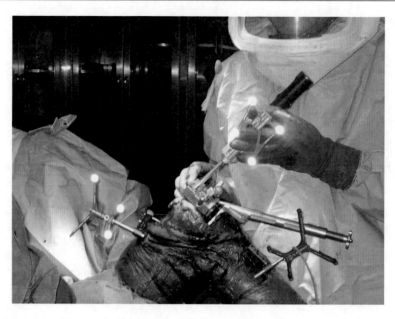

Fig. 15.1 Computer navigation in total knee arthroplasty using optical line-of-sight tracking, reflective balls on tracker, and LEDs on tracker

the tibial component in more than 3° of varus increased the odds of failure [4].

Computer-assisted alignment devices were developed to improve the positioning of implants during TKA. These systems include image-based and image-free navigation systems. Image-based systems use preoperative CT scans or operative fluoroscopic images to assist in implant positioning. Image-free navigation systems use information obtained in the operating suite with the aid of infrared probes (Fig. 15.1). Early data on the use of these systems appear positive with improved mechanical alignment, frontal and sagittal femoral axis alignment, and frontal tibial axis alignment. Furthermore, no studies have demonstrated increased complications compared with hand-guided techniques. Yau et al. compared the combined intraobserver error for image-free acquisition of reference landmarks during TKA, finding that the maximum combined error for the coronal plane mechanical axis alignment was 1.32° [5]. Bathis et al. compared an image-free navigation system with a conventional method using an intramedullary femoral guide and an extramedullary tibial guide. They reported the postoperative mechanical alignment to be within

3° varus or valgus in 96% of the navigation cases vs. 78% in the conventional group [6]. Sparmann et al. determined an image-free navigation system to produce a significant improvement in mechanical alignment, frontal and sagittal femoral alignment, and the frontal tibial alignment ($P<0.0001$) compared with a hand-guided technique. The postoperative mechanical alignment was within 3° varus or valgus in 87% of the conventional group vs. 100% of the navigation group [7].

Table 15.1 lists a number of recent studies that compare the use of imageless computer-assisted navigation with conventional methods for TKA. All studies are able to demonstrate a statistically significant improvement in terms of placing the final mechanical alignment of the knee within 3° of the ideal mechanical axis. Furthermore, we note that 94% of the overall cases reach this level of precision with computer navigation compared with 73% where conventional methods are used, and the difference does not change as the number of cases are accumulated from the various series.

There are other image acquisition and tracking methods beyond the current standard imageless total knee systems and these would include CT, fluoroscopy, and electromagnetic tracking.

Table 15.1 Recent publications comparing navigated with manual or conventional methods of determination of the mechanical axis compared to CAS

References	N	Navigated (%)	Manual (%)	% Difference
Haaker et al. (2005)	100	96	75	21
Sparmann et al. [7]	120	98	78	20
Victor and Hoste [9]	50	100	74	27
Jenny [15]	235	97	74	23
Jenny et al. (2001)	50	94	78	16
Kim et al. (2005)	69, 78	78	58	20
Perlick et al. (2004)	40	93	75	18
Song et al. (2005)	47, 50	96	76	20
Bathis et al. (2004)	160	96	78	18
Perlick et al. (2004)	50	92	72	20
Hart et al. (2003)	60	88	70	18
Oberst et al. (2006)	13	100	62	39
Anderson et al. (2005)	116, 51	95	84	11
		94	73 ($P < 0.001$)	20

Bathis et al. compared CT with imageless referencing methods in TKA, finding that 92% of CT vs. 97% with imageless referencing methods produced TKA mechanical axis alignment <3° [8]. Victor and Hoste used a fluoroscopic image acquisition in a randomized study with TKA to find 100% of navigated knees to have a mechanical alignment within ±2° while 73% of conventional TKAs were within ±2° [9]. Lionberger et al. compared electromagnetic trackers vs. optical line-of-site trackers in a prospective study using an imageless referenced TKA system, finding that 93% of cases with electromagnetic trackers had an alignment of <3° from the mechanical axis compared with 90% of cases where optical trackers were used [10].

Because of the recent popularity of electromagnetic trackers, a short discussion of accuracy issues is warranted. Lionberger et al. has studied the various facets of electromagnetic technologies, pointing out the important weaknesses of signal distortion from any conductive material and degradation of the signal by any ferrous or magnetic material. While software optimization has been developed with system lockout for various form of signal degradation, this has not been comprehensive enough to include materials such as copper or brass. In these examples, an error may be registered before the system can detect

abnormality. The working space for an electromagnetic coil is roughly a 30-cm cube. That means the tracking device or coil must remain within this limited space, and be held relatively rigid or still for appropriate signal acquisition. We have studied these factors in a simulated operating room setting for TKA, finding comparable accuracy with the standard optical line-of-sight system, with the caveat that unexplained "outliers" still occurred during testing (Fig. 15.2). We would caution that this technology, while promising, has not reached the industrial grade of precision present with most standard optical line-of-sight systems.

Blood loss has been shown to be significantly reduced with the use of computer navigation and avoidance of intramedullary rods. Kalairajah et al. were able to reduce the mean blood loss from 1,747 to 1,351 mL by using the pin-placed trackers instead of intramedullary guided femur and tibia jigs, which was a significant difference in 60 patients [11]. Kalairajah et al. performed a transcranial Doppler study on 14 patients, finding that all patients who had undergone intramedullary instrumentation of the femur and tibia with conventional TKA had documented intracranial microemboli compared with only 50% of those who had undergone procedures where only intracortical tracking pins had been placed [12].

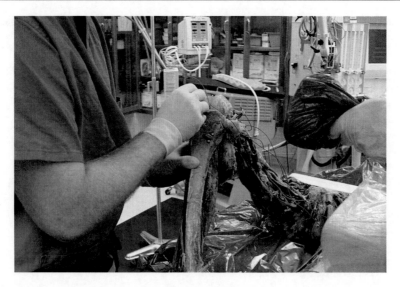

Fig. 15.2 Experimental registration using electromagnetic trackers for total knee arthroplasty

Unicondylar knee arthroplasty is a procedure that also may benefit from CAS. Cobb et al. used a computer-navigated robotic system to insert Oxford unicondylar knee implants, finding that, with CAS, all patients had the final implant placement within 2° of the planned position compared with 40% using conventional instruments [13]. Cossey et al. demonstrated that CAS-directed mechanical alignment for unicondylar arthroplasty was optimal in all cases while the conventional aligned cases had 4 of 15 cases where the axis was placed in the lateral joint compartment from mild overcorrection [14]. Jenny clearly demonstrated the improvement of unicondylar arthroplasty using navigation, both for a standard and a minimally invasive approach [15]. Keene et al. compared the results of conventional and CAS navigated unicondylar arthroplasties performed in bilateral cases, finding that 87% of navigated cases were within 2° of planned alignment compared with 60% of conventional cases [16].

Total Hip Arthroplasty

DiGioia et al. first described the use of CT for preoperative image acquisition subsequently utilized in the navigated surgical procedure [17]. This was done originally for acetabular component

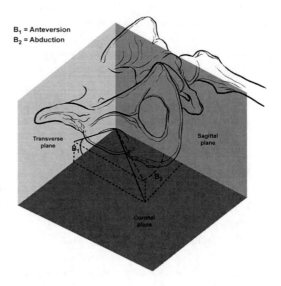

Fig. 15.3 Pelvic coordinate system used for standard measurement of cup inclination and anteversion with anterior pelvic plane

insertion. The other significant innovation was the description of the anterior pelvic plane as the baseline anatomical reference for measuring the position of the cup (Fig. 15.3). Several reports describe the accuracy of the cup placement in relation to the transverse axial plane to be 1°/1 mm. Haaker et al. compared the results of free-hand conventional instrumentation vs.

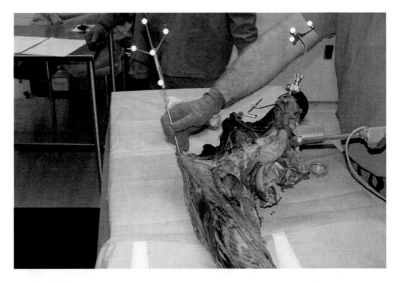

Fig. 15.4 Experimental registration of imageless total hip computer navigation system touch point marking the anterior superior iliac spine

CT navigation using postoperative CT for final evaluation in 98 patients. The target acetabular component position was 45° inclination and 20° anteversion. After CAS, average cup position was 43° abduction (95% confidence interval [CI]: 0.97) and 22.2° anteversion (95% CI: 1.72). For freehand, average cup position was 45.7° abduction (95% CI: 9.1°) and 28.5° anteversion (95% CI: 10.2°). The F ratio was 5.56 for abduction and 3.67 for ante-version ($P < 0.0001$) [18].

Imageless applications have been developed to eliminate the complexity and expense required for using CT. Kalteis et al. found that imageless referencing was comparable to CT navigation in a randomized and controlled trial [19]. Using the Lewinnek criteria of radiologic cup positioning to avoid dislocation of 40° inclination and 15° anteversion, 17% of CT navigated patients were outside the ±10° limits compared with 7% imageless navigation [20]. In that study, a "flip technique" was used for imageless referencing in the supine position and then repositioning to the lateral position. Nogler et al. attempted with cadavers to show an improvement over conventional acetabular cup positioning [21]. While a clear advantage was evident, the error was up to 8°, with a high standard deviation of 4.5° with the imageless method. Wixson et al. utilized CAS in patients who had undergone minimally invasive posterior

hip approaches for cup placement. At surgery, the mean values for inclination and anteversion in the CAS group were $42.38 \pm 1.88°$ (range 38–47°) and $20.78 \pm 2.58°$ (range 13–29°), respectively. They studied cup anteversion, finding that 30% of navigated cups were within a narrow range of 17–23° compared with only 6% of a manual control group.

While imageless methods of referencing have been advocated for total hip navigation, several authors have questioned the accuracy and precision of this approach. Stiehl et al. used several cadaver studies to evaluate cup positioning after imageless referencing [22] (Fig. 15.4). Using the imageless optical tracking referencing surgical navigation, mean acetabular inclination was 43.59° (standard deviation [SD] = 3.56°) and anteversion was 17.03° (SD = 1.01°). Their conclusion was that determination of cup inclination lacked precision, based on the relatively large standard deviation and range that was found. This was related in part to the relatively large area for touch point matching the anterior superior iliac spines. Another issue is the error created by the subcutaneous fat layer between skin and the bone landmarks, which has been determined to add 0.5° error for each millimeter of thickness.

Fluoroscopic referencing has been attempted as well for total hip arthroplasty, but suffers from

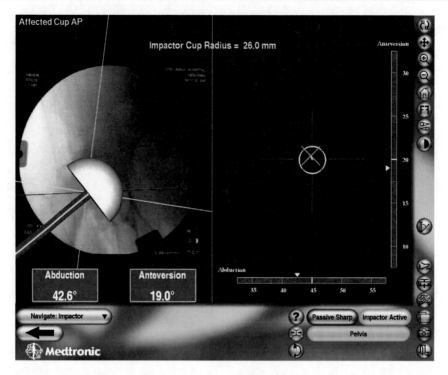

Fig. 15.5 Screen portrayal of fluoroscopic navigation of acetabular component, note projected inclination of 42° and anteversion of 19°

similar precision issues (Fig. 15.5). Most importantly, the field of vision of most standard fluoroscopy C-arms is limited to approximately 9 in. This makes image acquisition difficult, particularly if the patient is on the operating table. Stiehl et al. found that visualizing and referencing the pubic symphysis was problematic using fluoroscopy, leading to poor precision with cup anteversion [23] (Fig. 15.6). Cup inclination, on the other hand, was relatively accurate. Grutzner et al. has demonstrated significant improvements when fluoroscopy was combined with percutaneous touch pointing methods for determination of the anterior pelvic plane, perhaps rendering a more suitable system [24].

Pros

Total Knee Arthroplasty

Navigating a TKA has become my standard practice, beginning in September 2003, with now more than 250 cases completed. My hospital purchased the Medtronic Treon Stealth system, which uses optical cameras but has a variety of instruments and tracker options. The original "Universal Total Knee" software system was simple with excellent screen graphics and continues to be my software of choice. After experiencing several other examples, I think that any system to be of value for the surgeon must not add more than 5–15 min to the surgical procedure. From experience, I have developed a medial placement of the dynamic reference base (DRB) placing pins in the medial femoral transepicondylar axis and in the medial tibial shaft (Fig. 15.7). The idea is to have the frames located in the sagittal plane on the medial side of the leg, so that they are out of the way for all instrument placements, yet allowing easy access to the camera that is placed beyond the contralateral leg. Reference point matching is the critical step, and the most important points are the anterior femoral cortex (because I use an anterior cortical reference for the anterior-posterior cuts), femoral center, tibial center, and the distal malleoli (Fig. 15.8). In fact, the precision of any navigation system relies on

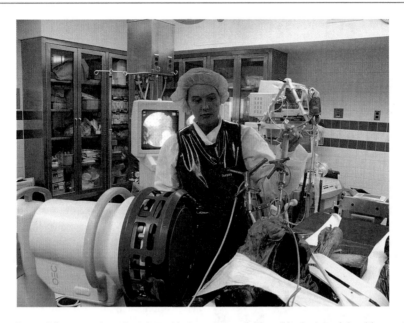

Fig. 15.6 Experimental fluoroscopic registration with the cadaver positioned in the lateral decubitus position

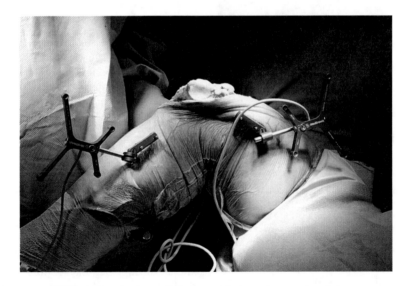

Fig. 15.7 Placement of LED trackers in the sagittal plane with femoral transepicondylar percutaneous position and medial tibial shaft percutaneous placement of dynamic reference bases

how accurately these points are referenced. The points of the procedure for which I rely almost solely on the computer are the initial ligament balancing, which is done in extension, tibial cut, distal femoral cut, anterior femoral cut, and gap measurements. With experience, one learns to rely on the computer for these measurements and will override positions suggested by conventional instruments.

A clinical study was done on my first 86 total knee cases comparing the final computer alignment readings with standing anteroposterior (AP) radiographs of the lower extremity, finding that 95% were within ±2° of the mechanical axis center line.

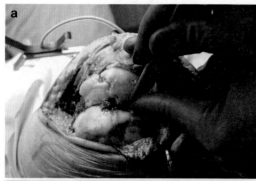

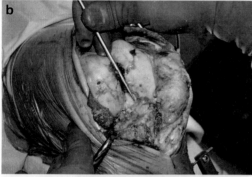

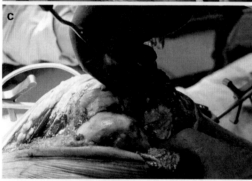

Fig. 15.8 (**a**) Touch point referencing of the femoral center, which is the bisection of the transepicondylar line and the anterior/posterior axis (Whiteside) line in total knee arthroplasty. (**b**) Touch point referencing of the femoral anterior/posterior axis, which also coincides with the tibial shaft axis in total knee arthroplasty. (**c**) Touch point referencing of the tibial center, which is the bisection of the transtibial axis

I found that other measurements, including the transepicondylar axis, Whiteside's AP axis, and the tibial rotational axes were too variable and of limited value in absolute terms. Joint line position reflected a resection amount within 1–2 mm of the healthy joint surface but required some judgment. Particular problems are best resolved with computer navigation. For example, any varus deformity greater than 10° from the

mechanical axis requires a ligament release that can be assessed by the computer (Fig. 15.9). I have learned that prior to surgical navigation, I was not fully releasing most of these knees. Stripping of the superficial collateral ligament is fairly extensive, going down 7–10 cm, and a "pop" of the medial ligament is needed to get the anatomical alignment. Similar findings are noted with valgus knee, where release will usually require a complete release of the iliotibial tract insertion, lateral capsule, and occasionally the femoral origin of the lateral collateral ligament. Old fracture deformities are best resolved with navigation (Fig. 15.10). Because femoral alignment is conventionally done with intramedullary instrumentation, bone blocks of the femoral canal usually require computer navigation for accurate assessment. Ligament-balancing measurements have become an important part of my techniques, and I strive for 1–2 mm laxity in full extension and less than 3 mm in flexion. This is done with gentle varus/valgus stresses throughout the range of motion. There are no practical instruments for assessing ligament balance currently available.

I have navigated ten failed total knees during revision TKA and found significant information in each case that subsequently guided the surgical technique. Several revisions have been done to correct chronic instability found after MIS "quadriceps-sparing" approaches. The typical problem is a residual varus deformity of 5–7°, which leaves the knee tight on the medial side in extension but lax on the lateral side in extension and on both sides in flexion. I have used the computer to correct the original deformity and then to appropriately balance the gaps, allowing for a simple exchange of a thicker polyethylene insert. The computer can also be used to define abnormal tibial and femoral component rotation that can be found with cases requiring revision for patella subluxation or dislocation.

Computer navigation has been an excellent intraoperative method to assess the precision and efficacy of newer MIS instruments (Fig. 15.11). I have found most of these nstruments to have a "toggle" or "wiggle" that easily translates into a 2-mm error. When performing MIS procedures, I heavily rely on the computer for all cuts, ligament release, and final measurements.

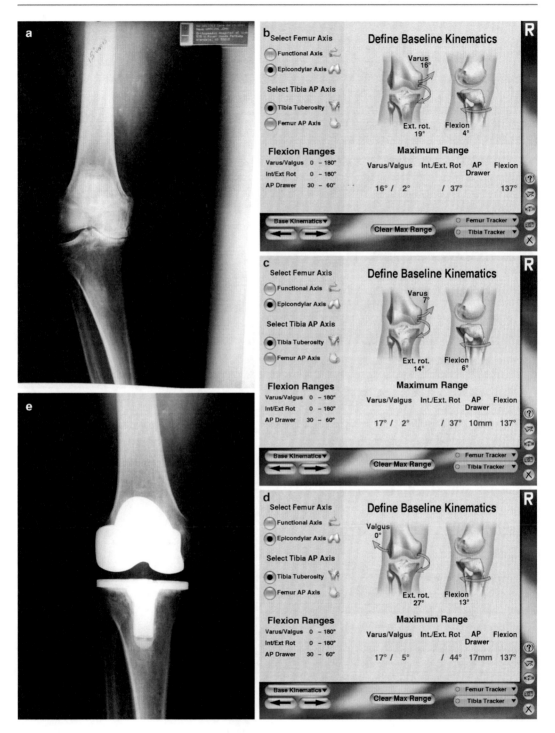

Fig. 15.9 (a) A 69-year-old man with a varus deformity that measures 16° from the mechanical axis. (b) Baseline screen shot on a computer demonstrates a 16° varus deformity. (c) Typical release with extensive stripping of the superficial medial collateral ligament and judged to be "adequate" by clinical experience is shown to be still in 7° of varus. (d) Further release to the point of "pop" of the superficial medial collateral ligament allows not for correction of 0° to the mechanical axis. (e) Postoperative AP standing radiograph shows correction with femorotibial axis of 6°

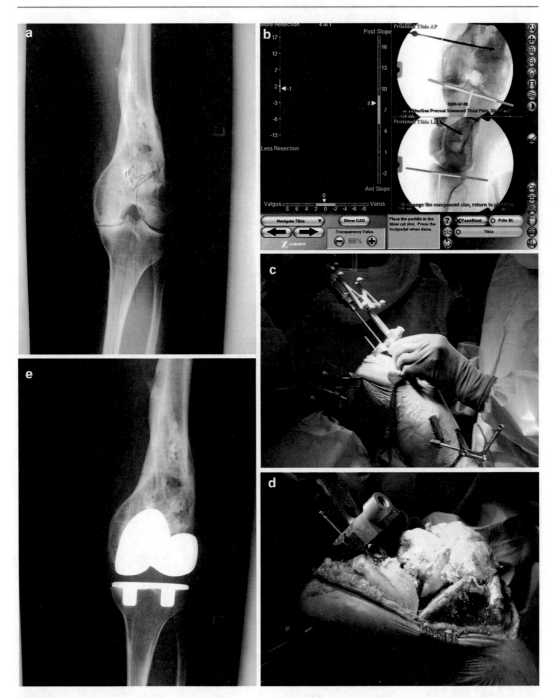

Fig. 15.10 (a) Difficult total reconstruction in an old distal femoral fracture deformity. (b) Navigation of tibial cut shows planned cut to be 8° posterior slope, 1 mm of medial tibial plateau, and 0° to the mechanical axis. (c) Freehand navigation of the distal femoral cutting guide into the desired resection level and correct angle for the coronal and sagittal planes. (d) The distal femoral cut is made based on the free-hand navigated position of the cut guide. (e) The final radiograph shows the "perfect" position of the distal femoral cut, with a final mechanical axis measurement of 1° varus

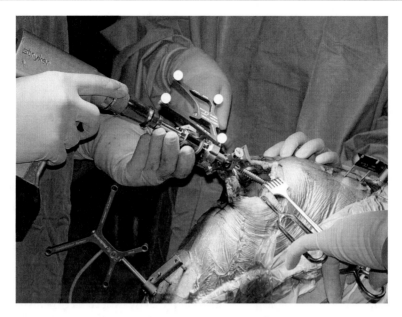

Fig. 15.11   Navigation of minimally invasive surgical distal femoral cut guide into the appropriate position

Total Hip Arthroplasty

The potential for satisfactory surgical navigation in total hip arthroplasty is very different from that in total knees. There is a suitable method for surgical navigation in total hips that has an accuracy approximating 1 mm/1°, but this requires the use of preoperative CT. Several studies have validated this fact. To date, there are no similar validations of imageless or fluoroscopic image acquisition techniques. Secondly, the primary applications for total hip arthroplasty have been for cup placement. Several new systems now offer the potential of determining femoral offset, femoral canal version, and leg length assessment. Most lack published scientific validation.

Cons

Total Knee Arthroplasty

The problems with computer navigation can be defined by two factors, increased cost and surgical time. Most early adopters have an advantage for costs because the benefits of the method can be marketed, increasing surgical case load. This

was clearly my situation, and I noted that patients were clamoring for the new technology. That stated, a typical capital system will cost the hospital $200,000, with the need of a maintenance contract of $20,000–$40,000 for software upgrades and other problems. This technology is in constant evolution requiring frequent adjustments. Surgical time is an important consideration and I would note that several current systems are cumbersome and time consuming. I have cut out all of the extra steps, doing only those things that I think are "value added" for my system. A typical case is lengthened only 7–10 min over the conventional approach.

For the community surgeon with lower surgical volume, purchasing a capital system may not be an option. Several companies now offer laptop systems that utilize innovative tracking methods such as the Zimmer Axiem electromagnetic system. The hospital rents the system on a per-case basis that closely approximates the cost of the typical capital system. Small electromagnetic trackers may be placed within the wound, avoiding the need for percutaneous pin placement. The disadvantage is the fact that any ferrous material, including instruments, operating table, etc. can degrade the accuracy of the system. In addition, an assistant must carefully position the magnetic coils to limit motion and to effectively collect the signal from the trackers. These problems limit the accuracy and efficacy of this technology.

A third factor that could be equated with costs is the expense of the "learning curve." This could require the surgeon and their staff to attend a surgical skill course to learn computer navigation. I personally spent several hours in the anatomy lab learning my system before performing live surgery. However, much effort has been made to create appropriate product literature to limit this process.

Total Hip Arthroplasty

Cost can be identified as the major drawback with total hip navigation and this carries all the problems noted above for total knees. The other serious reservation is time, and my experience with both the fluoroscopic and imageless systems has been that they are very time consuming. The current imageless applications require either a "flip technique" where the patient is moved from the supine to the lateral decubitus position, or a touch point matching method with the patient positioned in the lateral position. The point matching may be superficial or through percutaneous punctures. The "flip technique," although easy to perform, adds at least 15–20 min as a separate procedure. The reference base plate must be placed into position with percutaneous pins, the trackers must be attached with the quick release, and the optical camera positioned. After referencing, the tracker is removed, the patient is repositioned into lateral decubitus, and the pelvis and leg are prepped and draped for the formal total hip replacement. I have utilized fluoroscopic referencing for the lateral approach and virtually abandoned this approach. The field of view of the standard fluoroscopic C-arm is limited, making image acquisition challenging and time consuming. I think that these limitations will be resolved with new emerging technologies, such as intraoperative CT, that should allow for automated referencing and have a much larger field of view. Finally, any of these methods that use percutaneous

pin placement expose the patient to pin site infection, bone fracture, neuroma formation, or sensitive scar formation, although there are no reported cases to date of these problems.

Conclusions

CAS for total knee and hip arthroplasty has offered substantial improvements in the precision of the operative technique that should provide long-term benefits to the patient. In addition, the gains for minimally invasive surgery, although not proven, could be logically assumed. Optical systems for tracking are highly accurate and robust for this application. Electromagnetic tracking offers promise, although current systems are not presently as accurate. Total knee applications have evolved easily to an efficient imageless referencing protocol. Total hip applications remain cumbersome, and non CT-based systems lack the important precision that is needed. Significant improves loom on the horizon.

References

1. Bargar WL, Bauer A, Boerner M. (1998) Primary and revision total hip replacement using ROBODOC. Clin Orthop Relat Res Sep;(354):82–91
2. Jaramaz B, DiGioia AM III, Blackwell M, Nikou C. (1998) Computer assisted measurement of cup placement in total hip replacement. Clin Orthop Relat Res Sep;(354):70–81
3. Petersen T, Engh G. (1988) Radiographic assessment of knee alignment after total knee arthroplasty. J Arthroplasty 3:67–72
4. Berend M, Ritter M, Meding J, et al. (2004) Tibial component failure mechanisms in total knee arthroplasty. Clin Orthop Relat Res Nov;(428):26–34
5. Yau WP, Leung A, Chiu KY, Tang WM, Ng TP. (2005) Intraobserver errors in obtaining visually selected anatomic landmarks during registration process in nonimage based navigation-assisted total knee arthroplasty. J Arthroplasty 20:591–599
6. Bathis H, Perlick L, Tingart M, et al. (2004) Alignment in total knee arthroplasty. J Bone Joint Surg Br 86:682–687
7. Sparmann M, Wolke B, Czupalla H, et al. (2003) Positioning of total knee arthroplasty with and without navigation support. J Bone Joint Surg Br 85:830–835
8. Bathis H, Perlick L, Tingart M, et al. (2004) Radiological results of image-based and non-image-based

computer-assisted total knee arthroplasty. Int Orthop 28:87–90

9. Victor J, Hoste D. (2004) Image-based computer-assisted total knee arthroplasty leads to lower variability in coronal alignment. Clin Orthop Relat Res Nov;(428):131–139

10. Lionberger, DR. (2006) The attraction of electromagnetic computer navigation in orthopaedic surgery. In *Navigation and Minimally Invasive Surgery*, JB Stiehl, A Digioia, W Konermann, R Haaker (eds). Springer, Heidelberg

11. Kalairajah Y, Simpson P, Cossey AJ, Verrall GM, Spriggins AJ. (2005) Blood loss after total knee arthroplasty, effects of computer assisted surgery. J Bone Joint Surg Br 87:1480–1482

12. Kalairajah Y, Cossey AJ, Verall GM, Ludbrook G, Spriggins AJ. (2005) Are systemic emboli reduced in computer assisted surgery. J Bone Joint Surg Br 88:198–202

13. Cobb J, Henckel J, Gomes P, et al. (2006) Hands on robotic unicompartmental knee replacement. J Bone Joint Surg Br 88:188–197

14. Cossey AJ, Spriggins AJ. (2005) The use of computer-assisted surgical navigation to prevent malalignment in unicompartmental knee arthroplasty. J Arthroplasty 20:29–33

15. Jenny J-Y. (2005) Navigated unicompartmental knee replacement. Orthopaedics 28:1263–1267

16. Keene G, Simpson D, Kalairag Y. (2006) Limb alignment in computer assisted minimally-invasive unicompartmental knee replacement. J Bone Joint Surg Br 88:44–48

17. DiGioia AM, Jaramaz B, Plakseychuk AY, et al. (2002) Comparison of a mechanical acetabular alignment guide with computer placement of the socket. J Arthroplasty 17:359–364

18. Haaker R, Tiedjen K, Ottersbach A, Stiehl JB, Rubenthaler F, Shockheim M. (2007) Comparison of freehand versus computer assisted acetabular cup implantation. J Arthroplasty 22(2):151–159

19. Kalteis T, Handel M, Bathis H, Perlick L, Tingart M, Grifka J. (2006) Imageless navigation for insertion of the acetabular component in total hip arthroplasty. J Bone Joint Surg Br 88:163–167

20. Lewinnek GE, Lewis JL, Tarr R, et al. (1978) Dislocations after total hip-replacement arthroplasties. J Bone Joint Surg Am 60:217–220

21. Nogler M, Kessler O, Prassl A, et al. (2004) Reduced variability of acetabular cup positioning with use of an imageless navigation system. Clin Orthop Relat Res Sep(426):159–163

22. Stiehl JB, Heck DA. (2006) Validation of imageless total hip navigation. In *Navigation and Minimally Invasive Surgery in Orthopaedics*, JB Stiehl, A Digioia, W Konermann, R Haacker. (eds). Springer, Heidelberg

23. Stiehl JB, Heck DA, Jarmaz B, Amiot L-P. Comparison of fluoroscopic and imageless referencing in navigation of total hip arthroplasty. J Comput Assist Surg in press

24. Grutzner PA, Zheng G, Langlotz U, et al. (2004) C-arm based navigation in total hip arthroplasty – background and clinical experience. Injury 35(Suppl 1):A90

Minimally Invasive Total Knee Arthroplasty with Image-Free Navigation

16

S. David Stulberg

Computer-assisted surgery (CAS) is beginning to emerge as one of the most important technologies in orthopedic surgery. Many of the initial applications of this technology have focused on adult reconstructive surgery of the knee. The value of CAS in total knee arthroplasty (TKA) has been established in many studies. Minimally invasive surgical (MIS) techniques for performing TKA are also receiving extensive and intensive attention. The goals of this chapter are to (1) present the rationale for the use of image-free CAS in knee surgery, (2) explain the rationale for combining CAS with MIS techniques, (3) describe the basic components of an image-free navigation system, (4) illustrate a typical CAS MIS technique, and (5) present the initial results using this technique.

Rationale for the Use of Computer-Assisted Surgery in Knee Reconstruction

A successful surgical reconstruction of the knee requires proper patient selection, appropriate perioperative management, correct implant selection, and accurate surgical technique. The consequences of performing a knee reconstruction inaccurately have been well documented for total knee arthroplasties, unicondylar arthroplasties,

anterior cruciate ligament reconstructions, and high tibial osteotomies [1–35].

Although mechanical instrumentation has significantly increased the accuracy and reliability with which knee reconstructions are performed [36], errors in implant and limb alignment continue to occur, even when the procedures are performed by experienced surgeons. The accuracy with which these procedures are performed using manual instrumentation is dependent on the knowledge and experience of the surgeon and the frequency with which the surgeon performs the procedures.

Computer-assisted surgical techniques have been developed to address the inherent limitations of mechanical instrumentation [37–72]. The goals of integrating CAS with knee reconstruction techniques are to increase the accuracy of these procedures and reduce the proportion of alignment outliers that occur when these procedures are performed.

Errors in the alignment of bone resection can occur at numerous points during the performance of a knee reconstruction [73, 74]. The placement of the cutting blocks or ligament alignment jigs may be inaccurate. The attachment of these tools to bone may produce an error in their placement. The actual performance of the cut or drilling of the hole may be inaccurate (e.g., the saw blade may deflect). The final insertion of the implant may be inaccurate. Mechanical instrumentation does not provide a method for checking the accuracy of each of these steps of a knee reconstructive procedure. Integrating CAS with knee

S.D. Stulberg (✉)
Department of Orthopaedic Surgery, Feinberg School of Medicine, Northwestern University, Chicago, IL, USA
e-mail: jointsurg@northwestern.edu

G.R. Scuderi and A.J. Tria (eds.), *Minimally Invasive Surgery in Orthopedics: Knee Handbook*,
DOI 10.1007/978-1-4614-0679-2_16, © Springer Science+Business Media, LLC 2012

reconstruction allows the surgeon a means of placing cutting blocks accurately and measuring the accuracy with which each step of the procedure is performed. During the performance of an MIS TKA, visualization of each step of the procedure is difficult. Therefore, the ability to measure each step of the TKA procedure using CAS may be particularly important for MIS TKA [73–75].

The goal of knee reconstructive procedures is to align limbs and implants correctly. Restoration of appropriate kinematic relationships and ligamentous stability to the knee is also sought [76–78]. Mechanical instrumentation cannot measure the precision with which knee kinematics and ligament stability is restored. CAS techniques make it possible to determine the presurgical kinematic relationships and ligamentous stability of the knee and help guide the surgeon to restore the desired kinematic relationships and ligamentous balance.

Rationale for Combining MIS and CAS TKA Techniques

The rationale for an MIS TKA is that an accurate and properly executed TKA can be carried out safely using a surgical technique that may decrease the morbidity, accelerate the recovery, and improve the outcome of the surgical procedure.

MIS TKA exposures provide reduced visualization of critical surgical anatomy. This has led to the development of a number of modifications in the usual TKA procedure. The concept of a "mobile window" (visualization of a portion of the entire surgical field at any given time) has been described. Special retractors to enhance visualization have been developed. Instruments that are unique to less invasive surgery have been designed. A variety of exposures of the knee joint, including the subvastus, mid-vastus, and tri-vector, have been described in an attempt to optimize the goals of MIS TKA. In addition, the need for "assistants' choreography" (precise, atraumatic exposure by experienced personnel) has been emphasized.

The consequences of the reduced visualization associated with minimally invasive total knee exposures include: (1) implant malposition; (2) fracture of the femur, tibia, or patella; (3) neurovascular injuries; (4) compromised wound healing; and (5) prolonged operative time.

Computer-assisted techniques were developed to overcome the inherent limitations of manual instrumentation. The initial reports of performing TKAs with computer-assisted techniques using conventional, extensile surgical exposures indicate that increased accuracy of limb and implant alignment and reduced incidence of alignment outliers occurs [38, 67, 68, 77, 79–105]. Therefore, the rationale for combining computer-assisted and MIS techniques is that the reduction in perioperative morbidity and the improvement in early postoperative function that are achieved with less invasive exposures can be realized while retaining the accuracy of implant and limb alignment that can be achieved with computer techniques, even when crucial surgical anatomic landmarks are not visible.

The introduction of less invasive total knee surgical techniques has required the development of instruments and cutting guides that are compatible with smaller incisions and less extensile exposures. If computer-assisted techniques are to be applied to less invasive total knee procedures, the hardware, software, and navigation instruments must also be reconfigured for these reduced exposures. As the computer technologies are adapted to less invasive knee procedures, it is essential that they are: (1) safe; (2) accurate; (3) efficient; (4) cost effective; and (5) compatible with less invasive surgical sequences and tools. It is critical that the accuracy and safety associated with the use of computer-assisted technologies for total knee replacements performed using conventional exposures be retained when this technology is applied to less invasive knee replacement exposures. The accurate registration of critical anatomic landmarks must not be compromised when small incisions are used. Trackers and miniaturized navigated cutting blocks must remain securely fixed to bone during the performance of the less invasive procedures.

Hardware and Software Requirements for Surgical Navigation

A detailed description of the hardware and software needed to perform computer-assisted reconstructive knee surgery is beyond the scope of this chapter. However, it is important that knee surgeons understand the basic components of a computer-assisted orthopedic system so that they can use the system correctly, safely, and efficiently, and so that they can make intelligent choices regarding the appropriateness of various systems for their surgical needs.

The hardware devices common to CAS systems are: (1) imaging devices; (2) computers and the peripherals and interfaces to allow them to function in the operating room; and (3) localizers and trackers (Fig. 16.1a, b).

The imaging devices that are currently available for use with computer-assisted orthopedic

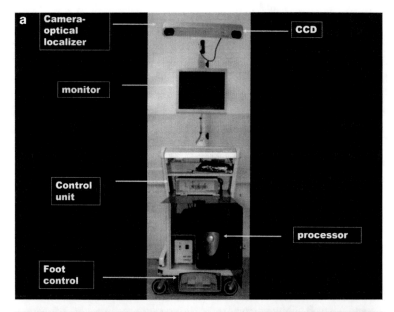

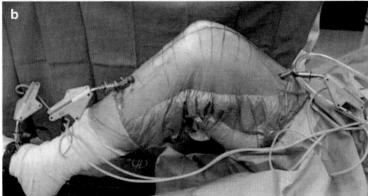

Fig. 16.1 (**a**) A typical image-free computer-assisted hardware system consisting of an optical tracker with charge-coupled devices (CCDs; the "cameras"), a computer monitor, control unit and processor, and a foot control system for communication between surgeon and the system. (**b**) Active trackers (also called rigid bodies or fiducials) attached to bicortical screws rigidly fixed to the femur and tibia

surgery systems include computed tomography (CT), magnetic resonance imaging (MRI), and fluoroscopy [42, 58, 62, 64, 79, 93–95, 106, 107]. These devices are used to acquire anatomical information on which a presurgical or intraoperative surgical plan is made. This plan becomes the basis for placing cutting tools intraoperatively and for establishing the alignment and stability of the knee. Although potentially extremely useful for knee reconstruction surgery, especially for robotic or customized surgery, imaging devices as currently employed with CAS knee systems have been perceived by surgeons as requiring additional and cumbersome steps to well-established knee procedures without providing significant benefits. Consequently, image-free computer-assisted systems have emerged as the most desired form of CAS for knee reconstruction.

A CAS knee navigation system can be thought of as an aiming device that enables real-time visualization of surgical action with an image of the operated structures. In order for this navigation to occur, it is necessary that the position and orientation of an instrument be visualized with respect to the anatomical structures to which it is attached. Therefore, contactless systems are used to communicate between the extremity and the computer system. Information can be transmitted using infrared light, electromagnetic fields, or ultrasound. Each method has its advantages and drawbacks. All of these methods allow several objects (e.g., two bones) to be viewed simultaneously.

The function of software in CAS systems is to integrate medical images and mathematical algorithms with surgical tools and surgical techniques [41, 42, 44]. A relatively small number of software components underlie most CAS image-free systems. These components include registration, navigation, procedure guidance, and safety.

Image-free CAS knee systems use as their preoperative plan concepts of limb and implant alignment that are currently used with manual instrumentation (e.g., restoration of the mechanical axis). In order to accomplish this plan, anatomic and kinematic information about a patient must be transmitted to the software on the computer and geometrically transformed using registration algorithms. Because bones are rigid and assumed unlikely to deform during the procedure, the algorithms used are termed *rigid*. These algorithms also require that the trackers attached to bones do not move during the procedure. Fiducial-based registration is a type of rigid registration. Therefore, the objects to which the LEDs are attached may be referred to as fiducials, trackers, or rigid bodies. Fiducial registration requires that at least three sets of markers be implanted into each bone or attached to each tool to determine the object's position and orientation. Therefore, each tracker must have at least three LEDs or reflecting spheres. Some CAS knee systems currently use shaped-based registration as an alternative to fiducial-based registration. These systems measure the shape of the bone surface intraoperatively and match the acquired shape to a surface model created from medical images and stored in the computer. The registration process for image-free knee navigation systems requires that information be acquired using kinematic techniques (e.g., circumducting the leg to determine the center of the femoral head) and/or surface registration techniques (e.g., touching bone landmarks with a probe).

Once the software takes anatomic and kinematic input from the extremity and geometrically transforms it, the surgeon is presented with a user interface that depicts, in sequence, the steps of the knee procedure. One of the most important objectives of software development in CAS knee surgery is to depict procedure sequences that are familiar to surgeons and with which they have become comfortable using manual instrumentation.

Example of an Image-Free, Minimally Invasive CAS Surgical Technique for TKA

Computer-assisted surgical technologies require that surgeons incorporate new tools into surgical routines with which they are experienced and comfortable. In fact, the most successful application

of CAS occurs when surgeons are very familiar with all aspects of the procedure in which CAS is used. Although the details of the CAS application for one knee procedure (e.g., TKA) vary from those of another knee procedure (e.g., anterior cruciate ligament [ACL] reconstruction), the basic principles and intraoperative steps are very similar for all of them. The TKA image-free navigation application is currently the most rapidly developing and most widely used CAS knee reconstruction technique. A brief description of a typical CAS MIS TKA will be described [69, 70, 107, 108].

Image-free CAS techniques do not require any special preoperative planning. The methods surgeons normally use to determine desired frontal and sagittal limb and implant alignment and implant sizes can be used to guide the intraoperative use of the CAS system. Mechanical alignment and CAS techniques use similar approaches for patient positioning and surgical exposure. Leg holders and pneumatic tourniquets that are routinely used with mechanical instrumentation can also be used with CAS.

The initial step in a TKA using CAS is the placement of the screws or pins in the distal femur and proximal tibia to which are attached the trackers (Fig. 16.1b). These are placed outside of the skin incision in a position that avoids injury to neurovascular structures and allows clear visualization of the trackers by the camera. Once the skin incision is made and the distal femur and proximal tibia are exposed, the anatomic landmarks critical for CAS-guided navigation are located. The center of the femoral head is determined using a kinematic registration technique (Fig. 16.2a, b). The hip is circumducted in a path guided by the visual cues displayed on the computer screen. The centers of the knee and ankle joint can be established using kinematic (Fig. 16.2c–f) or surface (Fig. 16.3a–i) registration techniques or a combination of both. The other anatomic landmarks located with a CAS probe are: (1) the distal femur (Fig. 16.3d, e); (2) the posterior condylar line (Fig. 16.3d, e); (3) the anterior femoral cortex (Fig. 16.3f); (4) the epicondylar axis; and (5) the medial and lateral tibial articular surfaces (Fig. 16.3g–i). The presurgical frontal and sagittal alignment, medial-lateral laxity in flexion and extension, and range of motion can then be measured and recorded (Fig. 16.4).

Both ligament balancing techniques (similar to those first described by Insall [13]) and anatomic approaches [12] can be used with CAS MIS TKA techniques. As with mechanically based techniques, the CAS anatomic procedures can begin with either the femoral or tibial preparation. In the example illustrated, the anatomic approach is used and the distal femur is resected first. A distal femoral cutting block with an attached tracker is placed on the anterior cortex of the femur. The proximal-distal, varus-valgus, and flexion-extension position of this block are guided by the CAS system (Fig. 16.5a, b). The CAS determination of femoral implant size and anterior-posterior placement can be made using either anterior or posterior referencing techniques. The rotation of the femoral component using CAS can be established using the posterior condylar line, the epicondylar line, or the patellar groove (Whitesides' line). A single navigation tool can be used to establish all of these femoral alignment and sizing objectives (Fig. 16.6a, b). The tibial cutting block, to which a tracker is attached, is placed in the desired position of varus-valgus and flexion-extension and at the desired resection level guided by the CAS system (Fig. 16.7a, b).

Once the femoral and tibial resections are completed, a trial reduction is carried out. The polyethylene insert that best balances the knee in flexion and extension is selected. The navigation system is used to measure the final alignment of the extremity, the amount of medial-lateral laxity in extension and flexion, and the final range of motion. The system can be used to guide the release of tight soft tissues medially, laterally, and posteriorly if this is necessary to establish a balanced, well-aligned knee. After the actual implants are inserted, the navigation system is used to measure the final frontal and sagittal alignment of the extremity, the final medial-lateral stability, and the final range of motion (Fig. 16.8).

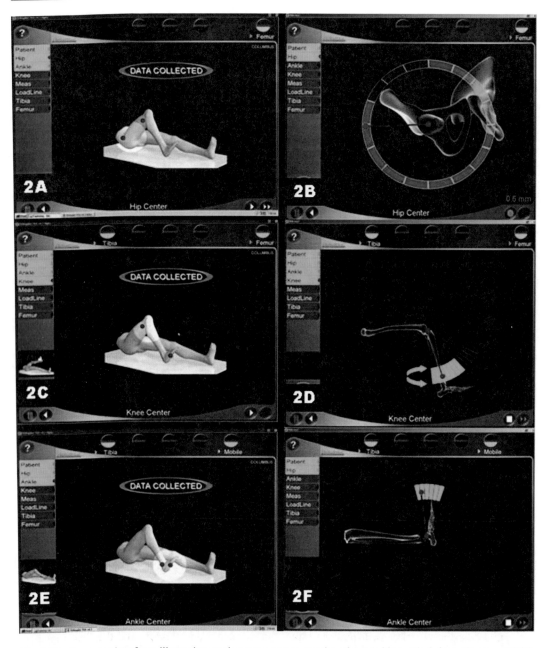

Fig. 16.2 Computer interfaces illustrating motion necessary to acquire adequate kinematic information to establish location of center of the (**a, b**) hip joint; (**c, d**) knee joint; and (**f, g**) ankle joint

Clinical Results of CAS MIS for Total Knee Arthroplasty

A prospective study was carried out to compare the effectiveness of CAS MIS TKA with manually performed MIS TKA.

Methods

Seventy-eight consecutive MIS TKA were performed by a single surgeon with extensive prior experience in both manual and CAS MIS TKA. Of the 78 TKA, 40 were performed ith

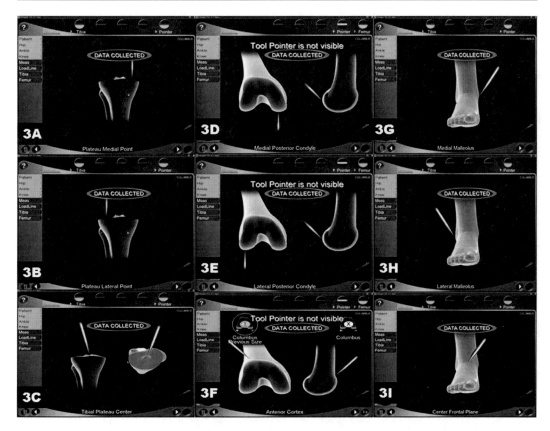

Fig. 16.3 Computer interfaces illustrating the position of the surface registration pointer necessary to acquire: (**a–c**) tibial medial and lateral articular surfaces and tibial mid-point; (**d–e**) the location of distal femoral articular surfaces and posterior condylar line; (**f**) the location of anterior femoral cortex; and (**g–i**) the location of center of ankle joint

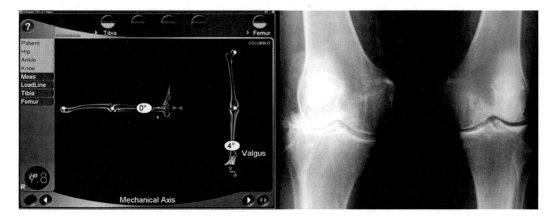

Fig. 16.4 Presurgical alignment depicted on the computer screen correlates with the alignment seen on the standing preoperative X-ray

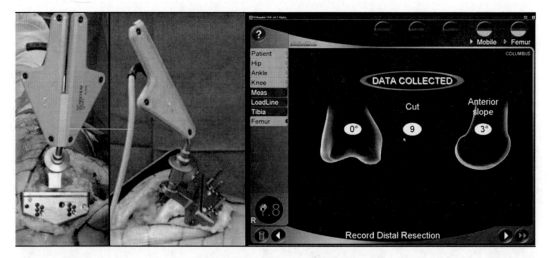

Fig. 16.5 Resection of a distal femur. (**a**) Frontal and sagittal position of a distal femoral cutting block with attached tracker. (**b**) Computer interface indicating the position of the distal femoral cutting block with regard to the frontal (0°) and sagittal (3° anterior slope) mechanical alignment and depth of resection (9 mm)

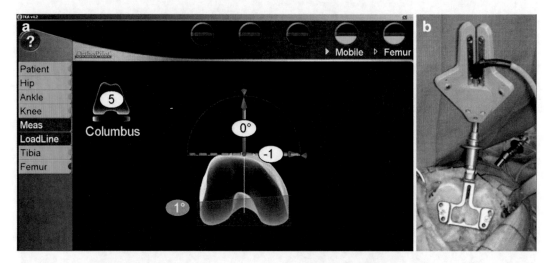

Fig. 16.6 Establishing position of four in one femoral cutting block. (**a**) Computer interface indicating rotation (0° relative to Whitesides' line) of the cutting block and anterior-posterior position of (in this case, the number 5) femoral component (1 mm above anterior cortex). (**b**) Navigation tool with attached tracker to establish rotation and anterior-posterior position of four in one femoral cutting block

MIS manual instruments and 38 with CAS MIS instruments. The groups were identical with regard to age, sex, body mass index (BMI), diagnosis, surgical technique, implants, and perioperative management. Preoperative and postoperative clinical examinations at 4 weeks, 6 months, and 1 year were performed by a physician blinded to the surgical techniques. Preoperative and postoperative radiographic measurements of the anterior-posterior mechanical axis and the sagittal tibial and femoral axes were evaluated by an observer blinded to the surgical technique. The Knee

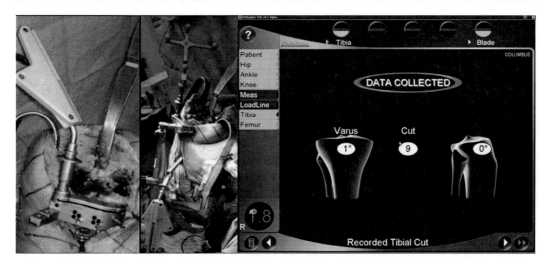

Fig. 16.7 Resection of a proximal tibia. (**a**) Frontal and sagittal position of a proximal tibial cutting block with attached tracker. (**b**) Computer interface indicating the position of the proximal tibial cutting block with regard to frontal (1° varus) and sagittal (0°) mechanical alignment and depth of resection from the least-involved tibial surface (9 mm)

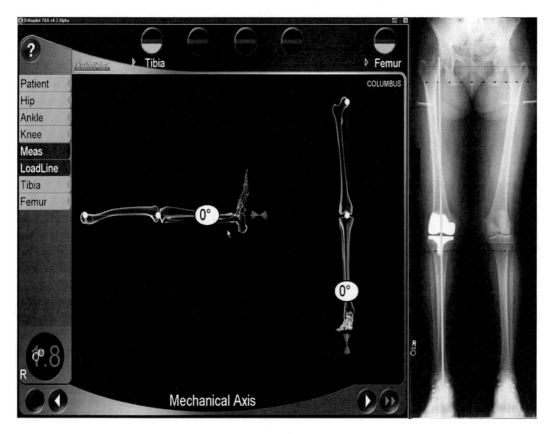

Fig. 16.8 Final frontal and sagittal alignment depicted on the computer screen correlates with the postoperative standing long X-ray

Table 16.1 Demographic data

	Unilateral manual	Unilateral CAS	Total
Number of patients	40	38	78
Age, in years (range)	64.0 (25.1–87.5)	65.7 (48.0–86.1)	64.8 (25.1–87.5)
Sex (% male)	43%	37%	40%
Diagnosis (% osteoarthritis)	100	100	100
BMI average (range)	31.5 (19.6–54.8)	33.9 (23.9–44.2)	32.7 (19.6–54.8)
Preoperative mechanical axis alignment (range); varus (+); valgus (−)	5.2 (−27 to 22)	8.9 (−12 to 20)	6.8 (−27to 22)
Preoperative knee score (range)	48.1 (17–77)	44.5 (22–79)	46.3 (17–79)
Preoperative function score (range)	56.7 (35–80)	50.4 (30–80)	53.6 (30–80)
Preoperative range of motion (range)	113.7 (70–140)	112.1 (70–140)	112.9 (70–140)
Preoperative pain calculation (range)	12.8 (0–30)	12.0 (0–45)	12.4 (0–45)

Society scoring system was used to assess clinical and functional outcomes relating to measures of range of motion, pain, knee stability, patient mobility, and movement independence (Table 16.1). Aesculap's Columbus cruciate-retaining, condylar implants were used in each patient. The Aesculap's OrthoPilot image-free navigation system was used for computer-assisted TKA. The study was approved by the Institutional Review Board of Northwestern University. The accuracy of the MIS manual instruments used by the surgeon at the beginning of his CAS experience has been previously reported [69].

Results

Clinical and functional scores were not significantly different between MIS CAS TKA and manual MIS TKA patients at 1 and 6 months postoperatively (Table 16.2). The average change in clinical and functional scores from preoperative to 1 and 6 months postoperative was also similar. Pain calculations were slightly higher (less pain) for CAS patients at 1 month postoperatively; however, no difference was noted at 6 months. Range of motion was not significantly different at 1 and 6 months postoperatively. The number of units of blood transfused was slightly greater for CAS patients and tourniquet time was on average, 27 min longer for CAS compared with manual TKA (Table 16.2). Mechanical axis, sagittal femoral axis, and sagittal tibial axis radiographic results were not significantly different (Table 16.3).

Discussion

Unlike the senior author's initial experience working with CAS [71, 103], this study found no statistically significant radiographic alignment differences between TKAs performed using CAS and manual techniques. This suggests either that external factors such as advancements in implants and mechanical alignment systems have resulted in manual TKA being performed more accurately, or that an improvement in the manual TKA technique has been realized through more than 4 years of extensive CAS utilization by the senior author. The MIS manual instruments used in this study were developed from alignment information obtained using image-free navigation techniques [37, 69, 73]. Although modifications in manual instrumentation can improve the accuracy with which MIS TKA can be performed, there are still have inherent limitations in the ability of this instrumentation to accurately determine the location of crucial alignment landmarks [37, 45]. Moreover, intraoperative measurements of the accuracy with which each step of a MIS TKA is performed can not be made with manual instrumentation. Many studies have demonstrated superior radiographic alignment outcomes with

Table 16.2 Selected variable results

	Unilateral manual			Unilateral CAS			Total		
	Average	Range	SD	Average	Range	SD	Average	Range	SD
Knee score[a] (preoperative)	48.1	(17, 77)	15.0	44.6	(22, 79)	13.7	46.3	(17, 79)	14.4
Knee score (1 month postoperative)	69.1	(40, 100)	14.3	75.4	(45, 98)	13.5	72.2	(40, 100)	14.1
Knee score (6 months postoperative)	84.6	(23, 100)	18.3	83.4	(32, 100)	18.5	84.0	(23, 100)	18.2
Function score' (preoperative)	56.7	(35, 80)	17.8	50.4	(30, 80)	12.2	53.6	(30, 80)	12.6
Function score (1 month postoperative)	48.9	(20, 100)	17.8	50.3	(20, 90)	14.9	49.6	(20, 100)	16.3
Function score (6 months postoperative)	62.0	(45, 90)	15.7	64.0	(30, 100)	19.4	62.9	(30, 100)	20.0
ROM (preoperative)	113.7	(70, 140)	15.7	112.1	(70, 140)	15.0	112.9	(70, 140)	15.3
ROM (1 month postoperative)	103.2	(65, 135)	13.5	105.1	(80, 125)	10.2	104.1	(65, 135)	11.9
ROM (6 months postoperative)	116.0	(100, 135)	8.7	117.0	(105, 135)	8.1	116.4	(100, 135)	8.4
Pain calculation[b] (preoperative)	12.8	(0, 30)	9.1	12.0	(0, 45)	9.7	12.4	(0, 45)	9.3
Pain calculation (1 month postoperative)	25.6	(10, 50)	12.5	29.3	(0, 50)	12.9	27.4	(0, 50)	12.8
Pain calculation (6 months postoperative)	39.5	(20, 50)	10.7	36.5	(0, 50)	15.6	38.1	(0, 50)	13.1
Units of blood transfused	0.4	(0, 4)	0.76	0.6	(0, 3)	0.82	0.48	(0, 4)	1.1
Tourniquet time (min)	72.9	(47, 110)	13.7	99.6	(60, 131)	16.3	85.1	(47, 147)	19.3
Mechanical axis (postoperative X-ray); Varus (+); Valgus (−)	−0.24	(−6, 8)	3.5	2.1	(−3, 7)	2.7	0.80	(−6, 8)	3.1
Femoral angle (postoperative)	2.6	(−6, 9)	3.2	2.2	(−2, 7)	2.2	2.5	(−6, 9)	2.6
Tibial angle (postoperative)	88.1	(83, 91)	1.7	88.0	(83, 92)	1.9	88.0	(83, 92)	1.8

[a]Best assessment = 100
[b]Maximum pain = 0; no pain = 50
SD standard deviation, ROM range of motion

CAS as compared with manual TKA. Therefore, the changes in the MIS mechanical alignment system do not seem sufficient to explain the equivalent alignment results obtained in this study.

This study suggests that it is also the intraoperative feedback and training effects realized through extensive use of a navigation system that has enabled the radiographic measures of manual MIS TKA to parallel those of CAS MIS TKA. It is possible for refinements in alignment perception, improvements in intraoperative judgment, and advances in technique to evolve to the point that no significant differences in radiographic alignment are apparent between CAS and manual TKA.

Clinical and patient-perceived functional results were not significantly different for CAS and manual TKA in this study. Outcome measures such as one's level of pain, range of motion, knee stability, mobility, and movement independence, which are measures of greatest importance to the TKA patient, were not significantly different in early follow-up. Thus, even if standard radiographs are not sensitive enough to detect subtle differences in alignment, these differences

Table 16.3 Variable change between preoperative, and 1- and 6-month follow-up

	Unilateral manual			Unilateral CAS			Total		
	Average	Range	SD	Average	Range	SD	Average	Range	SD
Knee score change; preoperative –1 month postoperative	20.9	(–18, 64)	21.3	30.8	(–15, 71)	20.6	25.8	(–18, 71)	21.4
Knee score change; preoperative – 6 months postoperative	36.7	(–26, 76)	26.0	36.9	(–6, 73)	25.7	36.8	(–26, 76)	25.5
Function score change; preoperative – 1 month postoperative	–4.4	(–40, 65)	21.0	–2.0	(–35, 55)	22.3	–3.2	(–40, 65)	21.4
Function score change; preoperative – 6 months postoperative	4.6	(–20, 35)	14.5	12.7	(–20, 30)	13.5	8.7	(–20, 35)	14.3
Range of motion change; preoperative – 1 month postoperative	–10.5	(–57, 38)	16.7	–4.7	(–48, 100)	24.4	–7.7	(–57, 100)	20.8
Range of motion change; preoperative – 6 months postoperative	3.3	(–15, 30)	11.6	8.1	(–87, 100)	36.1	5.5	(–87, 100)	25.7
Pain calculation change; preoperative – 1 month postoperative	12.8	(–20, 45)	13.7	17.4	(–25, 45)	15.2	15.1	(–25, 45)	14.6
Pain calculation change; preoperative – 6 months postoperative	25.5	(0, 50)	15.2	21.5	(–10, 50)	17.9	23.6	(–10, 50)	16.4

are not significant enough to influence short-term clinical and functional results. It is important to note the limitations of this study in terms of its duration. The long-term success of TKA is highly dependent on proper limb and implant alignment, thus, it is possible that alignment differences that were too minor to be exposed via standard radiograph in the short-term may become more readily apparent in long-term patient follow-up.

Summary

The widespread interest in minimally invasive arthroplasty surgery is focusing surgeons' attention on the importance of retaining accurate implant and limb alignment as exposure of surgical anatomy is reduced [75]. Techniques using nonfrontal resection planes (e.g., the "quadrant sparing" medial approach) are making clear how the position of an implant in one plane critically affects its position in all other planes [74]. CAS systems have the potential for greatly facilitating the evolution of MIS knee surgery. However, the CAS hardware and software must be configured to support safely, accurately, and efficiently the MIS systems that are being developed.

References

1. Aglietti P, Buzzi R. Posteriorly stabilized total-condylar knee replacement. J Bone Joint Surg 1988; 70-B(2):211–216
2. Ayers DC, Dennis DA, Johanson NA, et al. Common complications of total knee arthroplasty. J Bone J Surg 1997;2(79A):278–311
3. Bargren JH, Blaha JD, Freeman MAR. Alignment in total knee arthroplasty: correlated biomechanical and clinical observations. Clin Orthop Relat Res 1983 Mar;(173):178–183
4. Berger RA, Crosset LS, Jacobs JJ. Malrotation causing patellofemoral complications after total knee arthroplasty. Clin Orthop Relat Res 1998 Nov;(356): 144–153
5. Cartier P, Sanouillier JL, Frelsamer RP. Unicompartmental knee arthroplasty surgery. 10-year minimum follow-up period. J Arthroplasty 1996;11:782–788

6. Dorr LD, Boiardo RA. Technical considerations in total knee arthroplasty. Clin Orthop Relat Res 1986 Apr;(205):5–11

7. Ecker ML, Lotke PA, Windsor RE, et al. Long-term results after total condylar knee arthroplasty. Significance of radiolucent lines. Clin Orthop Relat Res 1987 Mar;(216):151–158

8. Fehring TK, Odum S, Griffin WL, Mason JB, Naduad M. Early failures in total knee arthroplasty. Clin Orthop Relat Res 2001 Nov;(392):315–318

9. Feng EL, Stulberg SD, Wixson RL. Progressive sub-luxation and polyethylene wear in total knee replacements with flat articular surfaces. Clin Orthop Relat Res 1994 Feb;(299):60–71

10. Goodfellow JW, O'Connor JJ. Clinical results of the Oxford knee. Clin Orthop Relat Res 1986 Apr;(205): 21–24

11. Hsu HP, Garg A, Walker PS, Spector M, Ewald FC. Effect on knee component alignment on tibial load distribution with clinical correlation. Clin Orthop Relat Res 1989 Nov;(248):135–144

12. Insall JW. Surgical approaches to the knee. In Insall JN (ed), *Surgery of the Knee*, Churchill Livingston, New York, 1984, pp. 41–54

13. Insall JN, Binzzir R, Soudry M, Mestriner LA. Total knee arthroplasty. Clin Orthop Relat Res 1985 Jan-Feb;(192):13–22

14. Insall JN, Ranawat CS, Aglietti P, Shine J. A compari-son of four models of total knee-replacement pros-thesis. J Bone Joint Surg 1976;58A:754–765

15. Jeffcote B, Shakespeare D. Varus/valgus alignment of the tibial component in total knee arthroplasty. Knee 2003;10(3):243–247

16. Jeffery RS, Morris RW, Denham RA. Coronal align-ment after total knee replacement. J Bone Joint Surg 1991;73B:709–714

17. Jiang CC, Insall JN. Effect of rotation on the axial alignment of the femur. Clin Orthop Relat Res 1989 Nov;(248):50–56

18. Laskin RS. Alignment of the total knee components. Orthopedics 1984;7:62

19. Laskin RS. Total condylar knee replacement in patients who have rheumatoid arthritis. A ten year follow-up study. J Bone Joint Surg 1990;72A: 529–535

20. Laskin RS, Turtel A. The use of an intramedullary tibial alignment guide in total knee replacement arthroplasty. Am J Knee Surg 1989;2:123

21. Nuno-Siebrecht N, Tanzer M, Bobyn JD. Potential errors in axial alignment using intramedullary instru-mentation for total knee arthroplasty. J Arthroplasty 2000;15:228–230

22. Oswald MH, Jacob RP, Schneider E, Hoogewoud H. Radiological analysis of normal axial alignment of femur and tibia in view of total knee arthroplasty. J Arthroplasty 1993;8:419–426

23. Petersen TL, Engh GA. Radiographic assessment of knee alignment after total knee arthroplasty. J Arthro-plasty 1988;3:67–72

24. Piazza SJ, Delp SL, Stulberg, SD, Stern SJ. Posterior tilting of the tibial component decreases femoral rollback in posterior-substituting knee replacement. J Orthop Res 1998;16:264–270

25. Ranawat CS, Boachie-Adjei O. Survivorship analy-sis and results of total condylar knee arthroplasty. Clin Orthop Relat Res 1988 Jan;(226):6–13

26. Rand JA, Coventry MB. Ten-year evaluation of geo-metric total knee arthroplasty. Clin Orthop Relat Res 1988 Jul;(232):168–173

27. Ritter MA, Faris PM, Keating EM, Meding JB. Postoperative alignment of total knee replacement. Its effect on survival. Clin Orthop Relat Res 1994 Feb;(299):153–156

28. Ritter M, Merbst WA, Keating EM, Faris PM. Radiolucency at the bone-cement interface in total knee replacement. J Bone Joint Surg 1991;76A:60–65

29. Sharkey PF, Hozack WJ, Rothman RH, et al. Why are total knee arthroplasties failing today? Clin Orthop Relat Res 2002 Nov;(404):7–13

30. Stern SH, Insall JN. Posterior stabilized prosthesis: results after follow-up of 9–12 years. J Bone Joint Surg 1992;74A:980–986

31. Teter KE, Bergman D, Colwell CW. Accuracy of intramedullary versus extramedullary tibial align-ment cutting systems in total knee arthroplasty. Clin Orthop Relat Res 1995 Dec;(321):106–110

32. Tew M, Waugh W. Tibiofemoral alignment and the results of knee replacement. J Bone Joint Surg 1985; 67B:551–556

33. Townley CD. The anatomic total knee: instrumenta-tion and alignment technique. The Knee: papers of the First Scientific Meeting of the Knee Society. Baltimore University Press, Baltimore, MD, 1985, pp. 39–54

34. Vince KIG, Insall JN, Kelly MA. The total condylar prosthesis. 10 to 12 year results of a cemented knee replacement. J Bone Joint Surg 1989;71B:93–797

35. Wasielewski RC, Galante JO, Leighty R, Natarajan RN, Rosenberg AG. Wear patterns on retrieved poly-ethylene tibial inserts and their relationship to techni-cal considerations during total knee arthroplasty. Clin Orthop Relat Res 1994 Feb;(299):31–43

36. Hungerford DS, Kenna RV. Preliminary experience with a total knee prosthesis with porous coating used without cement. Clin Orthop Relat Res 1983 Jun;(176):95–107

37. Currie J, Varshney A, Stulberg SD, Adams A, Woods O. The reliability of anatomic landmarks for deter-mining femoral implant=rotation in TKA surgery: implications for CAOS TKA. Presented at the Annual Meeting of Mid-America Orthopaedic Association, Amelia Island, FL, 2005

38. Delp SL, Stulberg SD, Davies B, Picard F, Leitner F. Computer assisted knee replacement. Clin Orthop Relat Res 1998 Sep;(354):49–56

39. Eichorn H.-J. Image-free navigation in ACL replace-ment with the OrthoPilot System. In Steihl JB, Konermann WH, Haaker RG (eds), *Navigation and Robotics in Total Joint and Spine Surgery*, Springer, Berlin, 2004, pp. 387–396

40. Ellis RE, Rudan JF, Harrison, MM. Computer-assisted high tibial osteotomies. In DiGioia AM,

Jaramaz B, Picard R, Nolte PL (eds), *Computer and Robotic Assisted Knee and Hip Surgery*, Oxford University Press, Oxford, 2004, pp. 197–212

41. Fadda M, Bertelli D, Martelli S, et al. Computer assisted planning for total knee arthroplasty. Proceedings of the First Joint Conference on Computer Vision, Virtual Reality and Robotics in Medicine and Medial Robotics and Computer Assisted Surgery, Grenoble, France. Springer, Berlin, 1997, pp. 619–628

42. Froemel M, Portheine F, Ebner M, Radermacher K. Computer assisted template based navigation for total knee replacement. North American Program on Computer Assisted Orthopaedic Surgery, 6–8 July 2001, Pittsburgh, PA

43. Garbini JL, Kaiura RG, Sidles JA, Larson RV, Matsen FA. Robotic instrumentation in total knee arthroplasty. 33 rd Annual Meeting, Orthopaedic Research Society, 19–22 January 1987, San Francisco, CA

44. Garg A, Walker PS. Prediction of total knee motion using a three-dimensional computer graphics model. J Biochem 1990;23:45–58

45. Jenny JY, Boeri C. Low reproducibility of the intra-operative measurement of the transepicondylar axis during total knee replacement. Acta Orthop Scand 2004;75(1):74–77

46. Julliard R, Lavallee S, Dessenne V. Computer assisted anterior cruciate ligament reconstruction of the anterior cruciate ligament. Clin Orthop Relat Res 1998 Sep;(354):57–64

47. Julliard R, Plaweski S, Lavallee S. ACL surgetics: an efficient computer-assisted technique for ACL reconstruction. In Steihl JB, Konermann WH, Haaker RG (eds), *Navigation and Robotics in Total Joint and Spine Surgery*, Springer, Berlin, 2004, pp. 405–411

48. Kaiura RG. Robot assisted total knee arthroplasty investigation of the feasibility and accuracy of the robotic process. Master's Thesis, Mechanical Engineering, University of Washington, Seattle, WA, 1986

49. Kienzle TC, Stulberg SD, Peshkin M, et al. A computer-assisted total knee replacement surgical system using a calibrated robot. Orthopaedics. In Taylor RH, et al. (eds), *Computer Integrated Surgery*. MIT Press, Cambridge, MA 1996, pp. 409–416

50. Kinzel V, Scaddan M, Bradley B, Shakespeare D. Varus/valgus alignment of the femur in total knee arthroplasty. Can accuracy be improved by pre-operative CT scanning? Knee 2004;11(3):197–201

51. Klos TVS, Habets RJE, Banks AZ, Banks SA, Devilee RJJ, Cook FF. Computer assistance in arthroscopic anterior cruciate ligament reconstruction. In DiGioia AM, Jaramaz B, Picard R, Nolte PL (eds), *Computer and Robotic Assisted Knee and Hip Surgery*, Oxford University Press, Oxford, 2004, pp. 229–234

52. Krackow K, Serpe L, Phillips MJ, et al. A new technique for determining proper mechanical axis alignment during total knee arthroplasty. Orthopedics 1999;22(7):698–701

53. Kuntz M, Sati M, Nolte LP, et al. Computer assisted total knee arthroplasty. International symposium on CAOS: 2000, February 17–19, Davos, Switzerland

54. Leitner F, Picard F, Minfelde R, et al. Computer-assisted knee surgical total replacement. First Joint Conference of CVRMed and MRCAS, Grenoble, France. Springer, Berlin, 1997, pp. 629–638

55. Leitner F, Picard F, Minfelde R, et al. Computer assisted knee surgical total replacement. Proceedings of the First Joint Conference on Computer Vision, Virtual Reality and Robotics in Medicine and Medical Robotics and Computer Assisted Surgery, Grenoble, France. Springer, Berlin, 1997, pp. 630–638

56. Martelli M, Marcacci M, Nofrini L, LA Palombara F, Malvisi A, Iacono F, Vendruscolo P, Pierantoni M. Computer- and robot-assisted total knee replacement: analysis of a new surgical procedure. Ann Biomed Eng 2000;28(9):1146–1153

57. Matsen FA, Garbini JL, Sidles JA. Robotic assistance in orthopaedic surgery. A proof of principle using distal femoral arthroplasty. Clin Orthop Relat Res 1993 Nov;(296):178–186

58. Nizard R. Computer assisted surgery for total knee arthroplasty. Acta Orthop Belg 2002;68(3):215–230. [Review]

59. Noble PC, Sugano N, Johnston JD, Thompson MT, Conditt MA, Engh CA Sr, Mathis KB. Computer simulation: how can it help the surgeon optimize implant position? Clin Orthop Relat Res 2003 Dec;(417):242–252. [Review]

60. Peterman J, Kober R, Heinze R, Frolich JJ, Heeckt PF, Gotzen L. Computer-assisted planning and robot assisted surgery in anterior cruciate ligament reconstruction. Oper Techn Orthop 2000;10:50–55

61. Picard F, Leitner F, Raoult O, Saragaglia D. Computer assisted knee replacement. Location of a rotational center of the knee. Total knee arthroplasty. International Symposium on CAOS, February 2000

62. Picard F, Moody JE, DiGioia AM, Jaramaz B, Plakseychuk AY, Sell D. Knee reconstructive surgery: preoperative model system. In DiGioia AM, Jaramaz B, Picard R, Nolte PL (eds), *Computer and Robotic Assisted Knee and Hip Surgery*, Oxford University Press, Oxford, 2004, pp. 139–156

63. Picard F, Moody JE, DiGioia AM, Martinek V, Fu FH, Rytel MJ, Nikou C, LaVarca RS, Jaramaz B. ACL reconstruction-preoperative model system. In DiGioia AM, Jaramaz B, Picard R, Nolte PL (eds), *Computer and Robotic Assisted Knee and Hip Surgery*, Oxford University Press, Oxford, 2004, pp. 213–228

64. Radermacher K, Staudte HW, Rau G. Computer assisted orthopaedic surgery with image-based individual templates. Clin Orthop Relat Res 1998 Sep;(354):28–38

65. Saragaglia D, Picard F. Computer-assisted implantation of total knee endoprosthesis with no preoperative imaging: the kinematic model. In Steihl JB, Konermann WH, Haaker RG (eds), *Navigation*

and *Robotics in Total Joint and Spine Surgery*, Springer, Berlin, 2004, pp. 226–233

66. Sati M, Staubli HU, Bourquin Y, Kunz M, Nolte LP. CRA hip and knee reconstructive surgery: ligament reconstructions in the knee-intra-operative model system (non-image based). In DiGioia AM, Jaramaz B, Picard R, Nolte PL (eds), *Computer and Robotic Assisted Knee and Hip Surgery*, Oxford University Press, Oxford, 2004, pp. 235–256

67. Siebert W, Mai S, Kober R, Heeckt PF. Technique and first clinical results of robot-assisted total knee replacement. Knee 2002;9(3):173–180

68. Stulberg SD, Eichorn J, Saragaglia D, Jenny J-Y. The rationale for and initial experience with a knee suite of computer assisted surgical applications. Third International CAOS Meeting, June, 2003, Marbella, Spain

69. Stulberg SD, Picard F, Saragaglia D. Computer assisted total knee arthroplasty. Operative techniques. Orthopaedics 2000;10(1):25–39

70. Stulberg SD, Saragaglia D, Miehlke R. Total knee replacement: navigation technique intra-operative model system. In DiGioia AM, Jaramaz B, Picard R, Nolte PL (eds), *Computer and Robotic Assisted Knee and Hip Surgery*, Oxford University Press, Oxford, 2004, pp. 157–178

71. Stulberg SD, Sarin V, Loan P. X-ray vs. computer assisted measurement techniques to determine pre and post-operative limb alignment in TKR surgery. Proceedings of the Fourth Annual American CAOS meeting, July 2001, Pittsburgh, PA

72. Tibbles L, Lewis C, Reisine S, Rippey R, Donald M. Computer assisted instruction for preoperative and postoperative patient education in joint replacement surgery. Comput Nurs 1992;10(5):208–212

73. Koyonos L, Granieri M, Stulberg SD. At what steps in performance of a TKA do errors occur when manual instrumentation is Used. Presented at the Annual Meeting of American Academy of Orthopaedic Surgeons, 2005, Washington, DC

74. Stulberg SD, Koyonos L, McClusker S, Granieri M. Factors affecting the accuracy of minimally invasive TKA. Presented at the Annual Meeting of American Academy of Orthopaedic Surgeons, 2005, Washington, DC

75. Tria AJ Jr. Minimally invasive total knee arthroplasty: the importance of instrumentation. Orthop Clin North Am 2004;35(2):227–234

76. Briard JL, Stindel E, Plaweski S, et al. CT free navigation with the LCS surgetics station: a new way of balancing the soft tissues in TKA based on bone morphing. In Steihl JB, Konermann WH, Haaker RG (eds), *Navigation and Robotics in Total Joint and Spine Surgery*, Springer, Berlin, 2004, pp. 274–280

77. Konermann WH, Kistner S. CT-free navigation including soft-tissue balancing: LCS-TKA and vector vision systems. In Steihl JB, Konermann WH, Haaker RG (eds), *Navigation and Robotics in Total Joint and Spine Surgery*, Springer, Berlin, 2004, pp. 256–265

78. Strauss JM, Ruther W. Navigation and soft tissue balancing of LCS total knee arthroplasty. In Steihl JB, Konermann WH, Haaker RG (eds), *Navigation and Robotics in Total Joint and Spine Surgery*, Springer, Berlin, 2004, pp. 266–273

79. Bathis H, Perlick L, Tingart M, Luring C, Perlick C, Grifka J.Radiological results of image-based and non-image-based computer-assisted total knee arthroplasty. Int Orthop 2004;28(2):87–90

80. Bohler M, Messner M, Glos W, Riegler ML. Computer navigated implantation of total knee prostheses: a radiological study. Acta Chir Aust 2000;33(Suppl):63

81. Clemens U, Konermann WH, Kohler S, Kiefer H, Jenny JY, Miehlke RK. Computer-assisted navigation with the OrthoPilot System using the search evolution TKA prosthesis. In Steihl JB, Konermann WH, Haaker RG (eds), *Navigation and Robotics in Total Joint and Spine Surgery*, Springer, Berlin, 2004, pp. 236–241

82. Jenny JY, Boeri C. Computer-assisted total knee prosthesis implantation without preoperative imaging. A comparison with classical instrumentation. Presented at the Fourth Annual North American Program on Computer Assisted Orthopaedic Surgery, 2000, Pittsburgh, PA

83. Jenny JY, Boeri C. Implantation d'une prothese totale de genou assistee par ordinateur. Etude comparative cas-temoin avec une instrumentaiton traditionnelle. Rev Chir Orthop 2001;87:645–652

84. Jenny JY, Boeri C. Navigated implantation of total knee prostheses: a comparison with conventional techniques. Z Orthop Ihre Grenzgeb 2001;139:117–119

85. Jenny JY, Boeri C. Unicompartmental knee prosthesis. A case-control comparative study of two types of instrumentation with a five year follow-up. J Arthroplasty 2002;17:1016–1020

86. Jenny JY, Boeri C. Unicompartmental knee prosthesis implantation with a non-image based navigation system. In DiGioia AM, Jaramaz B, Picard R, Nolte PL (eds), *Computer and Robotic Assisted Knee and Hip Surgery*, Oxford University Press, Oxford, 2004, pp. 179–188

87. Konermann WH, Sauer MA. Postoperative alignment of conventional and navigated total knee arthroplasty. In Steihl JB, Konermann WH, Haaker RG (eds), *Navigation and Robotics in Total Joint and Spine Surgery*, Springer, Berlin, 2004, pp. 219–225

88. Lampe F, Hille E. Navigated implantation of the Columbus total knee arthroplasty with the OrthoPilot System: Version 4.0. In Steihl JB, Konermann WH, Haaker RG (eds), *Navigation and Robotics in Total Joint and Spine Surgery*, Springer, Berlin, 2004, pp. 248–253

89. Mattes T, Puhl W. Navigation in TKA with the Navitrack System. In Steihl JB, Konermann WH, Haaker RG (eds), *Navigation and Robotics in Total Joint and Spine Surgery*, Springer, Berlin, 2004, pp. 293–300

90. Miehlke RK, Clemens U, Jens J-H, Kershally S. Navigation in knee arthroplasty: preliminary clinical experience and prospective comparative study in comparison with conventional technique. Z Orthop Ihre Grenzgeb 2001;139:1109–1129

91. Miehlke RK, Clemens U, Kershally S. Computer integrated instrumentation in knee arthroplasty: a comparative study of conventional and computerized technique. Fourth Annual North American Program on Computer Assisted Orthopaedic Surgery, Pittsburgh, PA, 2000, pp. 93–96

92. Nishihara S, Sugano N, Ikai M, Sasama T, Tamura Y, Tamura S, Yoshikawa H, Ochi T. Accuracy evaluation of a shape-based registration method for a computer navigation system for total knee arthroplasty. J Knee Surg 2003;16(2):98–105

93. Perlick L, Bathis H, Luring C, Tingart M, Grifka J. CT based and CT-free navigation with the brainLAB vector vision system in total knee arthroplasty. In Steihl JB, Konermann WH, Haaker RG (eds), *Navigation and Robotics in Total Joint and Spine Surgery*, Springer, Berlin, 2004, pp. 304–310

94. Perlick L, Bathis H, Tingart M, Perlick C, Grifka J. Navigation in total-knee arthroplasty: CT-based implantation compared with the conventional technique. Acta Orthop Scand 2004;75(4): 464–470

95. Perlick L, Bathis H, Tingart M, Kalteis T, Grifka J. [Usability of an image based navigation system in reconstruction of leg alignment in total knee arthroplasty – results of a prospective study] Biomed Tech (Berl) 2003;48(12):339–343. [German]

96. Picard F. Leitner F, Raoult O, Saragaglia D, Cinquin P. Clinical evaluation of computer assisted total knee arthroplasty. Second Annual North American Program on Computer Assisted Orthopaedic Surgery, Pittsburgh, PA, 1998, pp. 239–249.

97. Saragaglia D, Picard F, Chaussard C, et al. Computer-assisted knee arthroplasty: comparison with a conventional procedure: results of 50 cases in a prospective randomized study. Rev Chir Orthop Reparatrice Appar Mot 2001;87:215–220

98. Saragagaglia D, Picard F, Chaussard D, Montbarbon E, Leitner F, Cinquin P. Computer assisted total knee arthroplasty: comparison with a conventional

procedure. Results of 50 cases prospective randomized study. Presented at the First Annual Meeting of Computer Assisted Orthopaedic Surgery, Davos, Switzerland, 2001

99. Sparmann M, Wolke B. Knee endoprosthesis navigation with the Stryker System. In Steihl JB, Konermann WH, Haaker RG (eds), *Navigation and Robotics in Total Joint and Spine Surgery*, Springer, Berlin, 2004, pp. 319–323

100. Sparmann M, Wolke B. [Value of navigation and robot-guided surgery in total knee arthroplasty]. Orthopade 2003;32(6):498–505. [German]

101. Stockl B, Nogler M, Rosiek R, Fischer M, Krismer M, Kessler O. Navigation improves accuracy of rotational alignment in total knee arthroplasty. Clin Orthop Relat Res 2004 Sep;(426):180–186

102. Stulberg SD. CAS-TKA reduces the occurrence of functional outliers. Presented at the Annual Meeting of Mid-America Orthopaedic Association, Amelia Island, FL, 2005

103. Stulberg SD, Loan P, Sarin V. Computer-assisted navigation in total knee replacement: results of an initial experience in thirty-five patients. J Bone Joint Surg 2002;84-A(Suppl 2):90–98.

104. Wiese M, Rosenthal A. Bernsmann K. Clinical experience using the SurgiGATE System. In Steihl JB, Konermann WH, Haaker RG (eds), *Navigation and Robotics in Total Joint and Spine Surgery*, Springer, Berlin, 2004, pp. 400–404

105. Wixson RL. Extra-medullary computer assisted total knee replacement: towards lesser invasive surgery. In Steihl JB, Konermann WH, Haaker RG (eds), *Navigation and Robotics in Total Joint and Spine Surgery*, Springer, Berlin, 2004, pp. 311–318

106. Bathis H, Perlick L, Luring C, Kalteis T, Grifka J. [CT-based and CT-free navigation in knee prosthesis implantation. Results of a prospective study] Unfallchirurg 2003;106(11):935–940. [German]

107. Insall J, Scott N, Surgery of the knee, Chapter 95. Elsevier, Philadelphia, 2006, pp. 1675–1688

108. Mahfouz MR, Hoff WA, Komistek RD, Dennis DA. A robust method for registration of three-dimensional knee implant models to two-dimensional fluoroscopy images. IEEE Trans Med Imaging 2003;22(12): 1561–1574

The Utility of Robotics in Total Knee Arthroplasty

17

Mohanjit Kochhar and Giles R. Scuderi

In the last decade, instrumentation for total knee arthroplasty (TKA) has improved the accuracy, reproducibility, and reliability of the procedure. In recent years, minimally invasive surgery (MIS) TKA introduced instrumentation that was reduced in size to fit within the smaller operative field. As the operative field becomes reduced in size, the impact and influence of technology becomes proportionately larger [1]. The introduction of computer navigation with MIS is an attempt to improve the surgeon's visibility in a reduced operative field. The intended goal is to improve the position of the resection guides and ultimately the position of the final components, in essence, providing improved visualization in the limited field. This new technology is an enhancement tool or enabler in MIS TKA because, after registration of the anatomic landmarks, the instruments are dynamically tracked with real-time feedback on the angle and depth of the femoral and tibial resection. Currently, there are two types of computer-navigated systems for TKA: imaged-guided and imageless systems. Image-guided systems rely on data from preopera-

tive radiographs or computed tomography (CT) scans that are registered into the computer system. Imageless navigation systems eliminate the need for preoperative imaging and rely on the registration of intraoperative landmarks, and then compare the registered data with a library of anatomic specimens recorded within the computer databank. The next distinctive feature is the mode of instrument tracking, which can be either by optical line of sight with a series of arrays that are detected by an infrared camera, or an electromagnetic (EM) system that utilizes trackers that are attached to the bone and an EM field generator. Each computer navigation system has their proponents. Either way, advocates of computer-navigated surgery have reported in clinical studies that navigation has shown an improvement in the accuracy of component position within $3°$ of the desired position over conventional instrumentation [2, 3]. The computer relies on the registration of anatomic landmarks and interprets this data to create a three-dimensional (3D) virtual model of the knee. Refinements in the process of collecting the landmark data will create a more accurate virtual model and guidance system. The ideal system should be simple to use, accurate, and reliable without interfering with the operative field and should serve as an enabler in the limited operative field, reliably reporting the knee alignment and intraoperative kinematics [4].

Although it may be appealing to rely on computer navigation to perform a TKA, it is not artificial intelligence and does not make any of the surgical decisions. The procedure still is surgeon

M. Kochhar
North Middlesex University Hospital, London, UK

G.R. Scuderi (✉)
Insall Scott Kelly Institute for Orthopaedics and Sports Medicine, New York, NY, USA
e-mail: gscuderi@iskinstitute.com

North Shore-LIJ Health System, Great Neck, NY, USA

Albert Einstein College of Medicine, New York, NY, USA

directed, and navigation should serve as a tool of confirmation with the potential for improvements in surgical accuracy and reproducibility. Computer navigation is the first step in introducing advanced technologies into the operating room. The accuracy and safety of conventional instrumentation in TKA have always been dependent on the surgeon's judgment, experience, ability to integrate images, ability to utilize preoperative radiographs, knowledge of anatomic landmarks, knowledge of knee kinematics, and hand-eye coordination. Recent advances in medical imaging, computer vision, and robotics have provided enabling technologies. Synergistic use of computers and robotic technology, which are designed to develop interactive patient-specific procedures, optimize the accurate performance of the surgery [5]. The successful use of this technology requires that it not replace the surgeon, but support the surgeon with enhanced feedback, integration of information, and visual dexterity. The surgeon needs to clearly understand the goals, applications, and limitations of such a system [6].

TKA is ideally suited for the application of robotic surgery. The ability to isolate and rigidly fix the femur and tibia in known positions allows robotic devices to be securely fixed to the bone or within the desired plan of resection [7]. The bone is treated as a fixed object, simplifying the computer control of the robotic system. In developing the ideal robotic system, the technology must be safe; accurate; compatible with the operative field in size and shape, and be able to be sterilized; and must show measurable benefits, such as reduced operative time, reduced surgical trauma, and improved clinical outcomes [8]. Advocates think that this is attainable and that robotic-assisted TKA can achieve levels of accuracy, precision, and safety not accomplished by computer-assisted surgery [7].

The robotic systems rely on the creation of a 3D virtual model of the knee joint, which is formed from the identification of fixed anatomic landmarks. With all systems, the knee is rigidly secured in the same position with a leg-holding device throughout the referencing stage, as well as during the procedure to ensure accuracy. This establishes a relationship between the robot, the patient, and the surgical field. Using this information

and the created virtual model of the knee, the robot enables the surgeon to perform the guided surgery within a defined operative field. Commercially available robotic systems can be categorized as either passive or active devices. This classification is dependent on the control the surgeon has on the robot. With a passive system, the surgeon and robot interact and communicate during the procedure. While there is surgeon apprehension about active robots and automated surgery, passive systems that are in development may relieve the negative impression of robotics, the perception of increased risk, and potentially improve the surgeon's accuracy. A passive robotic system maintains surgeon control, which one does not want to relinquish, throughout the procedure. The surgeon selects the anatomic landmarks, which establishes the coordinate system that creates the virtual 3D model of the knee that guides the instrumentation. Surgeon input is preserved with confirmation of the implant size, the angle of resection, component rotation, and depth of resection. All of these factors can be adjusted prior to final positioning of the automated cutting guide. Once the cutting guide is guided into place, the surgeon resects the femur and tibia, as the surgeon would routinely do with standard instruments. Further concepts in development will provide intraoperative quantifiable information on soft tissue balancing, alignment, range of motion, and kinematics.

Passive robotic systems can be either with a haptic robot or a nonhaptic robot. With a haptic robot, a preoperative plan, established by the input of fixed bone landmarks, determines the boundaries of the surgical area. The tactile feedback with the cutting tool allows the surgeon to feel the boundaries of the bone resection and prevents movement outside of the planned operative field. Examples of this are the ACROBOT (Acrobot Co. LTD, United Kingdom) and the Haptic Guidance System (HGS) (MAKO Surgical Corp., Ft. Lauderdale, FL), which constrain the range of movement of the surgical tool held by a robotic arm. HGS is a haptic surgeon-assisted robotic system that allows the surgeon to accurately plan the implant size, and optimize the position and orientation of the implant relative to a CT scan acquired preoperatively. The system eliminates the need for cutting guides that are used in conventional knee arthroplasty. During the bone resection, the HGS system with its proprietary software continuously provides the surgeon with visual, tactile, and auditory guidance [9].

The nonhaptic robot assists the surgeon in accurately positioning the cutting guides based upon a preoperative plan and the recorded anatomic landmarks. The surgeon then performs the bone resection through the positioned cutting guide. There is no tactile feel to the resection, and the surgeon performs the resection through the cutting guide, as the surgeon would do with standard instrumentation. BRIGIT (Zimmer, Warsaw, IN) is a system in development that is an example of a passive robot. It is a multifunctional tool that serves as a passive assistant through an automated arm that positions and holds the resection guide according to the surgeon's surgical plan. The surgeon performs each step in the planned femoral and tibial resection for the desired knee implant as the robotic arm with the multifunctional cutting guide is positioned in place for each bone resection. The orientation and depth of resection is determined by the system software and confirmed by the surgeon. The bone resection is performed with a conventional saw. There is no tactile guidance during the bone preparation. The advantage of the robotic multifunctional cutting guide is that it eliminates the vast majority of instruments needed to perform the procedure, and the multifunctional cutting guide does not have to be pinned in place. It is locked in the plane of resection by the system during bone resection.

In contrast to a passive system, an active system follows a complete preoperative plan, which is carried out without surgeon intervention. After registration of the anatomic landmarks, the automated cutting tool resects the femur and the tibia. Examples of an active system are CASPAR (Universal Robot Systems, Germany) and ROBODOC (Integrated Surgical Supplies LTD, Sacramento, CA), which direct a milling device automatically according to preoperative planning [10]. These systems use preoperative CT images as part of the preoperative templating, including the angle and depth of bone resection, and the size of the components. After intraoperative registration of the anatomic landmarks, the computer matches this data with the CT scan and a virtual model of the knee is created. The surgeon then guides the robotic cutting tool to the desired location and the robot then prepares the bone autonomously. Upon completion of the bone preparation, the surgeon completes the TKA by balancing the soft tissues and implanting the components.

Robotic surgery is helping us take the next step into the operating room of the future. The role of robots in the operating room has the potential to increase as technology improves and appropriate applications are defined [1]. Joint replacement arthroplasty may benefit the most due to the need for high precision in placing instruments, aligning the limb, and implanting components. In addition, this technology will reduce the number of instruments needed for the procedure, improving efficiency. As technology advances, robots may be commonplace in the operating room and potentially transform the way TKA is done in the future. This is important because there has been an exponential rise in the number of TKA performed annually. With baby boomers coming of age, the rise in the number of people with arthritis and reported success of TKA in improving the quality of life, the number of TKA performed annually is rising. A recent report by Kurtz predicted that the number of primary TKA performed annually will increase to 3.48 million by 2030 [11]. This demand on surgeon and the hospital system will need improvements in technology in order to treat more patients and maintain the quality of care. Robotic surgery is new innovative technology and it will remain to be seen whether history will look on its development as a profound improvement in surgical technique or a bump on the road to something more important.

References

1. Scuderi GR. Smart tools and total knee arthroplasty. Am J Orthop 36(95)Supplement: 8–10, 2007
2. Alan RK, Shin MS, Tria AJ. Initial experience with electromagnetic navigation in total knee arthroplasty: a radiographic comparative study. J Knee Surg 20(2):152–157, 2007

3. Stiehl JB. Computer navigation in primary total knee arthroplasty. J Knee Surg 20(2):158–164, 2007
4. Scuderi GR. Computer navigation in total knee arthroplasty. Where are we and where are we heading. Am J Knee Surg 20(2):151, 2007
5. DiGioia AM, Jaramaz B, Colgan BD. Computer assisted orthopedic surgery. Image guided and robotic assistive technologies. Clin Orthop Relat Res 354:8–16, 1998
6. Specht LM, Koval KJ. Robotics and computer assisted orthopedic surgery. Bull Hosp Jt Dis 60:168–172, 2001
7. Adili A. Robotic assisted orthopedic surgery. Semin Laparosc Surg 11(2):89–98, 2004
8. Hurst KS, Phillips R, Viant WJ, etal. Review of orthopedic manipulator arms. Stud Health Technol Inform 50:202–208, 1998
9. Roche M. Changing the way surgeons plan and execute minimally invasive unicompartmental knee surgery. Orthopedic Product News July/August 2006
10. Surgano N. Computer assisted orthopedic surgery. J Orthop Sci 8(3):442–448, 2003
11. Kurtz S, Ong K, Lau E etal. Projection of primary and revision hip and knee arthroplasty in the United States 2005–2030. J Bone Joint Surg 89A:780–785, 2007

Electromagnetic Navigation in Total Knee Arthroplasty

18

Rodney K. Alan and Alfred J. Tria Jr.

Accurate limb alignment in total knee arthroplasty (TKA) is an essential part of the reconstructive procedure. Good alignment has been shown to correlate with improved outcomes. Malalignment of components greater than 3–4° may be associated with early failure [1–7]. The goal of computer-assisted TKA is to improve alignment. Theoretically, improved alignment should decrease the incidence of failure due to surgical technique.

Traditionally, intramedullary and extramedullary guides have been used to facilitate accurate bone cuts in TKA. Intramedullary alignment guides have been shown to have a high level of accuracy for the femur, but are less accurate for the tibia because the intramedullary canal does not always allow easy insertion of the reference rods [8–14]. Intramedullary guides align the limb relative to the anatomic axis. When using intramedullary guides, most surgeons cut the distal femur between 4° and 7° of anatomic valgus. Unlike conventional TKA, navigated TKA references the mechanical axis. With navigated TKA, the mechanical axis is more likely to show less

variation postoperatively [4, 15–25]. Slotted cutting guides have also been used to help to control the saw blade to increase bone cutting accuracy [26]. With the advent of computer-assisted surgery, slotted cutting guides can be positioned by navigation. This technique has been used effectively to improve the accuracy of alignment relative to the mechanical axis. Multiple studies have shown that postoperative alignment is improved using computer-assisted navigation when compared with performing TKA with conventional alignment guides [4, 15–25, 27]. Based on these studies, computer-assisted navigation in TKA may lead to improved outcomes.

Two types of navigation systems are available for TKA: image-assisted navigation and image-free navigation. Image-assisted techniques require radiographic studies to complete the procedure. Preoperative computed tomography (CT) scans or intraoperative fluoroscopic images are used by the computer as a reference for the anatomy. Image-assisted navigation increases the amount of time and planning required for performing navigated TKA and also exposes the patient to radiation.

Many navigation systems have transitioned into image-free techniques. The advantage of image-free navigation is the elimination of preoperative or intraoperative imaging. Image-free navigation requires kinematic localization of the hip center in order to identify the alignment of the limb.

Optical (or line-of-sight) navigation systems are available as image assisted and image free. With line-of-sight navigation, placement of optical

R.K. Alan
Department of Surgery, Saint Peter's University Hospital, New Brunswick, NJ, USA

A.J. Tria Jr. (✉)
Institute for Advanced Orthopaedic Study, The Orthopaedic Center of New Jersey, Somerset, NJ, USA
e-mail: atriajrmd@aol.com

Department of Orthopedic Surgery, Robert Wood Johnson Medical School, Piscataway, NJ, USA

G.R. Scuderi and A.J. Tria (eds.), *Minimally Invasive Surgery in Orthopedics: Knee Handbook*, DOI 10.1007/978-1-4614-0679-2_18, © Springer Science+Business Media, LLC 2012

tracking units (arrays) is detected by an infrared camera. All of the current studies on computer-assisted navigation in TKA use the line-of-site technique [4, 15–25].

Electromagnetic (EM) navigation is different from optical navigation. With EM technology, small dynamic referencing frames (DRF) are attached to the femur and the tibia within the operative exposure (Fig. 18.1), and a small hand-held electromagnetic emitter is used to track the DRFs (Fig. 18.2).

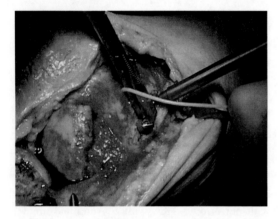

Fig. 18.1 The femoral DRF is attached to the medial metaphyseal bone

Advantages and Disadvantages of EM Navigation

EM navigation does not require a line-of-sight. The emitter sets up a field around the DRFs and the instruments. The computer can see the devices in the field and relate them to known anatomic landmarks identified by the surgeon. The emitter eliminates the need for the camera and the difficulties of lining the camera up with the reflective spheres of the arrays. The line-of-sight arrays required percutaneous pin fixation to the underlying femur and tibia. This exposes the knee to possible stress fracture through the pin holes and can lead to persistent drainage with the possibility of associated infection. The DRFs take the place of the arrays and are attached to the bone with small cortical screws.

Metal interference is a major problem with EM navigation. In the clinical setting, if there is too much interference, there is no image on the computer screen. It is possible that minor interference will still allow tracking but decrease the accuracy of the measurements [28]. The DRFs must be placed in a protected area in the knee so that no instruments change the position of the

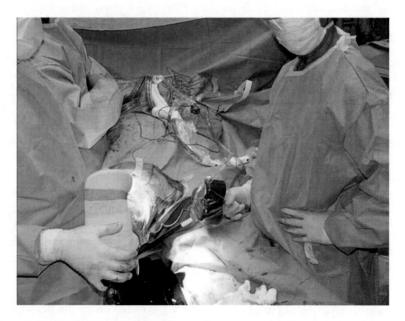

Fig. 18.2 The emitter is handheld with a sterile cover over it

sensing devices. The DRFs presently have wires that are attached to the computer, and these wires sometimes interfere with the surgical exposure. If the wire is cut, the DRF must be replaced and all of the land marking must be repeated.

Patients with cardiac pacemakers should not have EM navigation unless their pacemaker has been approved for use with EM navigation. The vendor who provides the device also provides a list of approved cardiac pacemakers that do not preclude EM navigation.

The kinematic hip center registration does require motion of the hip on the ipsilateral side to the TKA. The most recent software for EM navigation requires approximately 15° of abduction and adduction and 10° of combined internal and external rotation to localize the hip center. Thus, if the hip is fused, the EM navigation will not be possible. The emitter should be placed in a firm holding base for the kinematic centering of the hip because slight motion delays the process and sometimes invalidates the result. During the remainder of the operative procedure, the emitter can be handheld.

Technique

EM navigation can be used with any surgical approach for TKA. The technique does not require any change in the preparation of the case or in the surgical draping. All of the steps for EM navigation are carried out during the surgical procedure within the operative field. EM navigation requires the computer, the emitter, some retractors with decreased iron content, and the disposables. The disposables are sterile and include a registration stylus, a paddle probe, one DRF for the femur, one DRF for the tibia, and small screws for securing the referencing frames. The emitter and disposables should be connected prior to making the incision.

The DRFs are positioned and secured on the femur and the tibia after making the initial approach to the knee. Extensive soft tissue releases should be avoided until the initial alignment is recorded with the navigation. The placement of the DRFs is important because any motion of the referencing frames will diminish

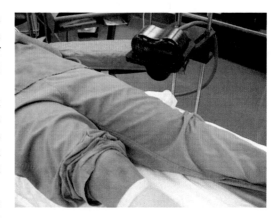

Fig. 18.3 The emitter holder attaches to the operating table and holds the device stable for navigation of the hip center (Innovative Medical Products, Plainville, CT, USA)

the accuracy of navigation. The referencing frames should be placed away from the areas of the bone that may be disturbed by the saw blade or broaches or instruments. The femoral referencing frame should be placed on the medial aspect of the femur at least 2 cm above the joint line, and the tibial referencing frame should be placed on the medial aspect of the tibia at least 1.5 cm below the joint line. The instruments are closest to the femoral DRF during the anterior resection of the femoral cortex. The tibial DRF is at greatest risk during the intramedullary broaching for the tibial stem.

After placing the DRFs, kinematic registration of the hip center can be completed. The EM field should be large enough so that the DRFs will remain in the field for approximately 15° of abduction and adduction and 10° of combined internal and external rotation of the limb. It is essential that there is no motion in the emitter or the pelvis during localization of the hip center. An emitter holder attached to the operating room table expedites the process (Fig. 18.3). The land marking of the knee is completed using the disposable pointer probe.

Throughout the remainder of the operative procedure, the navigation can be used to make the primary cuts or to check the cuts after they are completed with traditional instrumentation. It is best to use a mixture of both approaches until the surgeon is familiar with the technique. The EM monitoring can be used for the femoral rotation and the alignment in the coronal and sagittal planes. The tibial cut can also be monitored in the coronal and sagittal planes but the software is not currently able to evaluate the axial rotation of the component.

The patella is prepared in standard fashion without the aid of computer navigation. With the trial components in position, the laxity of the knee can be tested with the EM monitoring in full extension and 90° of flexion. Displacement of 2 mm or less with stress testing is ideal.

The final alignment and range of motion can be confirmed after the final components are inserted. The DRFs are disposable, but the authors have used the referencing frame in the contralateral knee on bilateral procedures without any difficulty.

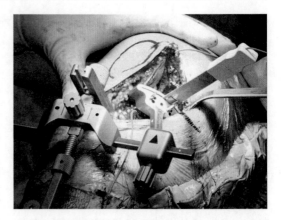

Fig. 18.4 The EM paddle is placed into the cutting slot of the extramedullary tibial guide for direct referencing of the cut

Materials and Methods

After obtaining institutional review board (IRB) approval, 60 consecutive patients who underwent TKA with EM navigation were reviewed. The navigation was used to measure the preoperative and postoperative alignment, and to confirm the cuts during the procedure. A standard intramedullary femoral alignment guide was used to make the distal femoral resection, and a modified extramedullary alignment guide was used to resect the proximal tibia (Fig. 18.4). After each bone resection, the paddle was used to measure the alignment of the cut (Fig. 18.5).

Preoperative and postoperative X-rays were used to measure the coronal plane alignment of the knee and the alignment of the tibial component. All X-rays were taken with the same technique. The knee was in full extension with the patella directed perpendicular to the X-ray beam [29].

The radiographic alignment of the knee was compared with the EM navigated alignment of the knee, using 6° of anatomic valgus as neutral for radiographs, and a mechanical axis of zero as neutral for EM navigation. Paired differences between X-ray and EM measures of alignment were generated to determine the relationship between radiographic

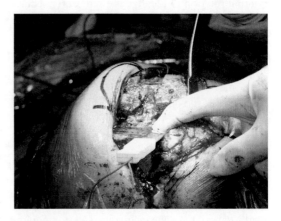

Fig. 18.5 The EM paddle is placed onto the cut surface of the tibia to recheck the cut

alignment measured on a 14 × 17-in. cassettes and EM-navigated alignment.

A separate analysis with another consecutive series of 20 patients was completed using preoperative and postoperative mechanical axis radiographs. Paired differences were analyzed to assess the relationship between mechanical axis radiographs and EM navigation.

Results

In the initial experience, EM navigation was abandoned in three operative procedures. On one occasion, the technical problem was solved by replacing the emitter. In another case, one of the DRFs was slightly loose and the computer began generating abnormal data. A wire was incidentally cut during one procedure.

When compared with anatomical alignment measured on short radiographs, the alignment measured by EM was within 3° of the predicted preoperative alignment in 63% (33/52) of cases. The alignment measured by EM was within 3° of the predicted postoperative alignment in 67% (38/57) of cases. The alignment of the tibial component measured by EM was within 3° of the predicted postoperative X-ray alignment in 87% (48/55) of cases.

When compared with mechanical axis radiographic alignment, the alignment measured by EM was within 3° of the predicted preoperative alignment in 90% (18/20) of cases. The postoperative alignment was within 3° in 90% (18/20) of cases; and the tibial component position was within 3° in 95% (19/20) of cases.

Discussion

Improvement of alignment during TKA and avoiding the potential concerns of optical navigation systems prompted the authors to investigate EM navigation. The technique is not difficult and can be adapted in a step-wise fashion until the surgeon becomes proficient with the system. Although the referencing frame and the wires are in the operative exposure, careful technique can eliminate the concern for cutting them during the procedure. The average tourniquet time was 69 min for the entire operative procedure in the author's initial experience with EM navigation. There were no surgical delays due to interruption in camera line-of-sight and no difficulties with debris interfering with arrays. There were no major complications. In three cases where the computer malfunctioned or the DRF was disturbed, the surgeries were completed with standard instrumentation.

The relationship between radiographic alignment and EM alignment was evaluated to determine the accuracy of EM navigation. Although there is some inherent variability in X-ray measurements, [30, 31] it is currently the standard for

evaluating limb alignment after TKA [8–14]. The maximum difference between the alignment demonstrated by EM navigation and alignment measured by mechanical axis radiographs was 4.2°. The mean differences are within 3° in 89% of cases. Two degrees may be the limit of what can be measured by X-rays; [32] therefore, EM navigation appears to be accurate.

When compared with anatomical alignment measured on short X-rays, the maximum difference can be as high as 9° when neutral is considered to be 6° of anatomic valgus. Many surgeons continue to use short X-rays to evaluate the results of TKA. Extraarticular deformity such as bowing is commonly not seen on short radiographs [33]. This causes the anatomic alignment to vary relative to the mechanical alignment. Six degrees of anatomic valgus is not neutral in all patients [34]. Surgeons who use navigation and rely on short radiographs only should be aware of the variability of the anatomical axis after navigated TKA.

The assumption of some articles regarding navigation is that the alignment determined by the computer is absolutely accurate [35]. This assumption is not entirely correct and the operating surgeon must be aware of the limitations of any system that is used for operative support. All systems that rely on kinematic hip center determination may have some error in assessing alignment. Victor and Hoste reported a mean deviation between the kinematic and radiographic hip center of 1.6 mm with a range of 0–5 mm [25]. They also suggested that other systems may have even more variability. Anatomical landmark registration is also a source for computer error. It is sometimes difficult to accurately identify all of the anatomic landmarks that are necessary for navigation [36]. Motion in the referencing frames adversely effects computer measurement of alignment and anatomic variation makes it difficult for any one software program to calculate the alignment correctly on every occasion. Finally, navigated alignment is determined with the knee joint in the non-weight-bearing position on the operating room table with the patella subluxated laterally and with a portion of the deep medial collateral ligament released as a part of the surgical approach. The radiographs are taken with the knee in the weight-bearing position and without any opening or laxity of the capsule. These factors can contribute to differences in alignment when measured by navigation and X-rays.

Conclusions

EM navigation for TKA can be adopted for clinical use with a short learning curve. The system appears to be accurate within 1 or 2°, comparable to optical navigation. The pitfalls of metallic interference and DRF motion are not difficult to surmount. Navigation is, in general, a supportive tool that can improve the accuracy of TKA but it must also be monitored throughout the operative procedure.

References

1. Bargren JH, Blaha JD, Freeman MA. Alignment in total knee arthroplasty. Correlated biomechanical and clinical observations. Clin Orthop Relat Res 1983 Mar;(173):178–83
2. Hvid I, Nielsen S. Total condylar knee arthroplasty. Prosthetic component positioning and radiolucent lines. Acta Orthop Scand 1984 Apr;55(2):160–5
3. Jeffery RS, Morris RW, Denham RA. Coronal alignment after total knee replacement. J Bone Joint Surg Br 1991 Sep;73(5):709–14
4. Kim SJ, MacDonald M, Hernandez J, Wixson RL. Computer assisted navigation in total knee arthroplasty: improved coronal alignment. J Arthroplasty 2005 Oct;20(7 Suppl 3):123–31
5. Lotke PA, Ecker ML. Influence of positioning of prosthesis in total knee replacement. J Bone Joint Surg Am 1977 Jan;59(1):77–9
6. Ritter MA, Faris PM, Keating EM, Meding JB. Postoperative alignment of total knee replacement. Its effect on survival. Clin Orthop Relat Res 1994 Feb;(299):153–6
7. Wasielewski RC, Galante JO, Leighty RM, Natarajan RN, Rosenberg AG. Wear patterns on retrieved polyethylene tibial inserts and their relationship to technical considerations during total knee arthroplasty. Clin Orthop Relat Res 1994 Feb;(299):31–43
8. Bono JV, Roger DJ, Laskin RS, Peterson MG, Paulsen CA. Tibial intramedullary alignment in total knee arthroplasty. Am J Knee Surg 1995 Winter;8(1):7–11
9. Cates HE, Ritter MA, Keating EM, Faris PM. Intramedullary versus extramedullary femoral alignment systems in total knee replacement. Clin Orthop Relat Res 1993 Jan;(286):32–9
10. Dennis DA, Channer M, Susman MH, Stringer EA. Intramedullary versus extramedullary tibial alignment systems in total knee arthroplasty. J Arthroplasty 1993 Feb;8(1):43–7
11. Evans PD, Marshall PD, McDonnell B, Richards J, Evans EJ. Radiologic study of the accuracy of a tibial intramedullary cutting guide for knee arthroplasty. J Arthroplasty 1995 Feb;10(1):43–6
12. Ishii Y, Ohmori G, Bechtold JE, Gustilo RB. Extramedullary versus intramedullary alignment guides in total knee arthroplasty. Clin Orthop Relat Res 1995 Sep;(318):167–75
13. Reed SC, Gollish J. The accuracy of femoral intramedullary guides in total knee arthroplasty. J Arthroplasty 1997 Sep;12(6):677–82
14. Teter KE, Bregman D, Colwell CW Jr. The efficacy of intramedullary femoral alignment in total knee replacement. Clin Orthop Relat Res 1995 Dec;(321):117–21
15. Anderson KC, Buehler KC, Markel DC. Computer assisted navigation in total knee arthroplasty: comparison with conventional methods. J Arthroplasty 2005 Oct;20(7 Suppl 3):132–8
16. Bathis H, Perlick L, Tingart M, Luring C, Perlick C, Grifka J. Radiological results of image-based and non-image-based computer-assisted total knee arthroplasty. Int Orthop 2004 Apr;28(2):87–90. Epub 2004 Jan 17
17. Bathis H, Perlick L, Tingart M, Luring C, Zurakowski D, Grifka J. Alignment in total knee arthroplasty. A comparison of computer-assisted surgery with the conventional technique. J Bone Joint Surg Br 2004 Jul;86(5):682–7
18. Bolognesi M, Hofmann A. Computer navigation versus standard instrumentation for TKA: a single-surgeon experience. Clin Orthop Relat Res 2005 Nov;440:162–9
19. Chauhan SK, Scott RG, Breidahl W, Beaver RJ. Computer-assisted knee arthroplasty versus a conventional jig-based technique. A randomized, prospective trial. J Bone Joint Surg Br 2004 Apr;86(3):372–7
20. Decking R, Markmann Y, Fuchs J, Puhl W, Scharf HP. Leg axis after computer-navigated total knee arthroplasty: a prospective randomized trial comparing computer-navigated and manual implantation. J Arthroplasty 2005 Apr;20(3):282–8
21. Hankemeier S, Hufner T, Wang G, Kendoff D, Zheng G, Richter M, Gosling T, Nolte L, Krettek C. Navigated intraoperative analysis of lower limb alignment. Arch Orthop Trauma Surg 2005 Aug;12:1–5
22. Matsumoto T, Tsumura N, Kurosaka M, Muratsu H, Kuroda R, Ishimoto K, Tsujimoto K, Shiba R, Yoshiya S. Prosthetic alignment and sizing in computer-assisted total knee arthroplasty. Int Orthop. 2004 Oct;28(5):282–5. Epub 2004 Aug 14
23. Perlick L, Bathis H, Tingart M, Perlick C, Grifka J. Navigation in total-knee arthroplasty: CT-based implantation compared with the conventional technique. Acta Orthop Scand 2004 Aug;75(4):464–70

24. Sparmann M, Wolke B, Czupalla H, Banzer D, Zink A. Positioning of total knee arthroplasty with and without navigation support A prospective, randomized study. J Bone Joint Surg Br 2003 Aug;85(6): 830–5

25. Victor J, Hoste D. Image-based computer-assisted total knee arthroplasty leads to lower variability in coronal alignment. Clin Orthop Relat Res 2004 Nov;(428):131–9

26. Plaskos C, Hodgson AJ, Inkpen K, McGraw RW. Bone cutting errors in total knee arthroplasty. J Arthroplasty 2002 Sep;17(6):698–705

27. Stockl B, Nogler M, Rosiek R, Fischer M, Krismer M, Kessler O. Navigation improves accuracy of rotational alignment in total knee arthroplasty. Clin Orthop Relat Res 2004 Sep;(426):180–6

28. Stiehl JB. Comparison of imageless and electromagnetic referencing protocols in total knee arthroplasty. Presented at the closed meeting of The Knee Society, September, 2006

29. Hall-Rollins J. Lower limb. In: Bontrager KL (ed.) Textbook of Radiographic Positioning and Related Anatomy. St. Louis, MO: Mosby;2001, p. 231

30. Lonner JH, Laird MT, Stuchin SA. Effect of rotation and knee flexion on radiographic alignment in total knee arthroplasties. Clin Orthop Relat Res 1996 Oct;(331):102–6

31. Swanson KE, Stocks GW, Warren PD, Hazel MR, Janssen HF. Does axial limb rotation affect the alignment measurements in deformed limbs? Clin Orthop Relat Res 2000 Feb;(371):246–52

32. Laskin RS. Alignment of total knee components. Orthopedics 1984;7:62–72

33. Petersen TL, Engh GA. Radiographic assessment of knee alignment after total knee arthroplasty. J Arthroplasty 1988;3(1):67–72

34. Hsu RW, Himeno S, Coventry MB, Chao EY. Normal axial alignment of the lower extremity and load-bearing distribution at the knee. Clin Orthop Relat Res 1990 Jun;(255):215–27

35. Stulberg D. How accurate is current TKR instrumentation? Clin Orthop Relat Res 2003 Nov;(416):177–84

36. Robinson M, Eckhoff DG, Reinig KD, Bagur MM, Bach JM. Variability of landmark identification in total knee arthroplasty. Clin Orthop Relat Res 2006 Jan;442:57–62

Robotics in Total Knee Arthroplasty

19

Werner Siebert, Sabine Mai, and Peter F. Heeckt

Total knee arthroplasty (TKA) has become the standard procedure in the management of degenerative joint disease after conservative therapy options have been exhausted. However, despite conscientious planning and carefully performed procedures, surgeons are often unsatisfied with implant alignment. Various authors described significant axial or rotational malalignment, and mediolateral and ventrodorsal tilt [1–4]. Seemingly small displacements of 2.5 mm potentially alter the range of motion by as much as 20° [5]. None of the contemporary improvements in implant design and instrumentation has alleviated these problems.

This led to the development of various robotic systems for improved precision in surgery. Robots are able to accurately position and move tools, thereby reducing human error. These systems rely on preoperative imaging, registration, and planning. The first clinical use was reported 1985 in the field of neurosurgery [6]. Orthopedic surgeons started using robotic devices around 1992 for total hip arthroplasty [7]. The active surgical robot CASPAR® (Computer-Assisted Surgical Planning and Robotics) was adapted for total hip and knee arthroplasty and for anterior cruciate ligament repair [8]. The first robot-assisted knee

replacement with this system was performed in March of 2000 in the Orthopedic Center Kassel. A total of 108 consecutive cases were operated on at this institution and followed-up for at least 5 years in a prospective study [9].

Surgical Technique

Robot-assisted TKA consists of the placement of fiducial markers, computed tomographic (CT) scanning, preoperative planning, and surgery.

Placement of Fiducial Markers

To facilitate orientation, the robot requires placement of a femoral and a tibial pin that serve as fiducial markers for each bone (Fig. 19.1). The robot uses these pins for spatial orientation and performs geometric calculations based on their location.

CT Scanning and Preoperative Planning

A helical CT scan is obtained immediately after the pins have been placed. Particular attention is paid to the areas of the femoral head, the pins, the knee, and the ankle. The CT data are then transferred into the PC-based planning station. The technical quality of the scan is automatically

W. Siebert (✉) • S. Mai
Kassel Orthopaedic Center, Kassel, Germany
e-mail: werner.siebert@vitos-okk.de

P.F. Heeckt
Smith & Nephew, Inc, Memphis, TN, USA

G.R. Scuderi and A.J. Tria (eds.), *Minimally Invasive Surgery in Orthopedics: Knee Handbook*,
DOI 10.1007/978-1-4614-0679-2_19, © Springer Science+Business Media, LLC 2012

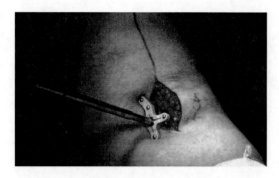

Fig. 19.1 Fastening of the special CT cross on the tibial pin (From Konermann W, Haaker R (eds.), Navigation und Robotic in der Gelenkund Wirbelsäulenchirurgie. Berlin, Springer, 2003, with kind permission of Springer Science + Business Media, Inc.)

checked and the pin position is verified. The surgeon identifies specific anatomical landmarks. The anatomical and mechanical axes of the femur and tibia are then calculated in the frontal and sagittal planes. The joint line, epicondylar twist, torsion of the tibia, as well as the relationship of the dorsal part of the tibia and the condylar line serve as additional important parameters. All angles and possible geometric translations are displayed on the video screen at the end of the planning procedure (Fig. 19.2).

The system allows the user to select and position a specific implant in different sizes. Unintentional notching can easily be avoided.

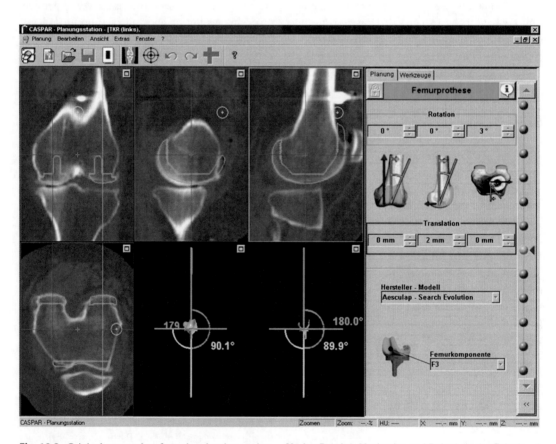

Fig. 19.2 Original screen-shot from the planning station showing the PC-based planning of the femoral component and the resulting mechanical leg axis (From Konermann W, Haaker R (eds.), Navigation und Robotic in der Gelenkund Wirbelsäulenchirurgie. Berlin, Springer, 2003, with kind permission of Springer Science + Business Media, Inc.)

With computer-assisted planning, the strong interdependence of all parameters, including the mechanical axes, becomes quite evident. Implant fit can be accurately assessed by scrolling through the scan. The system informs the user about the expected change in "extension" and "flexion gaps" and the resulting ligament tension. After positioning the implants, it is important to specify the milling areas in order to avoid redundant cutting and to protect the surrounding soft tissue. As a last step, the system prints out an overview of the final plan. All data are stored on a PC card and transferred to the robot control unit immediately before surgery.

Robot-Assisted Surgery

A conventional median incision with parapatellar approach to the knee joint is used. The knee joint is secured by a transfemoral and transtibial self-cutting screw to a specially designed frame. This rigid frame is also used for fixation of self-holding soft tissue retractors. In order to control for unwanted micro-movements of the leg during robotic surgery, rigid bodies with light-emitting diodes (LEDs) are firmly attached to the frame. The LED signal is constantly monitored by an infrared camera system, which will automatically shut off the robot in the event of excessive motion (Fig. 19.3). After registration of the fiducial markers, robotic milling is started by the surgeon. The cutting tool is equipped with internal water cooling and irrigation. A splash guard helps to keep the operative field and LEDs dry and clean (Fig. 19.4). Milling heads are changed during the procedure depending on the type of cut to be made. Varying with the size of the implant and bone density, the entire milling procedure takes approximately 18 min. If required, it is possible to revert to conventional manual technique at any point during surgery.

The resulting bone surfaces are accurately shaped and smooth (Fig. 19.5). After the fixation frame and pins are removed, soft tissues are balanced and the components of the implant are inserted. In this study, we started with the

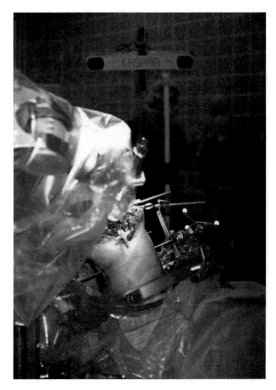

Fig. 19.3 View of the working robot. Unwanted motion is detected by an infrared camera system as seen in the background and corresponding rigid bodies fixed to the frame in the foreground (From Konermann W, Haaker R (eds.), Navigation und Robotic in der Gelenkund Wirbelsäulenchirurgie. Berlin, Springer, 2003, with kind permission of Springer Science + Business Media, Inc.)

cemented LC Search Evolution knee system (Aesculap, Tuttlingen, Germany) in the robotic group because this was the first knee implant system geometry that was loaded into the planning software.

Patients and Methods

A total of 108 knees were operated on using the robot system CASPAR. The following cruciate-retaining implant designs were used: 70 Search Evolution (Aesculap), 31 PFC Sigma® (DePuy Orthopedics, Inc., Warsaw, IN), and 7 Genesis (Smith & Nephew, Memphis, TN). Of these, 55 were implanted with both components being cemented (Figs. 19.6a, b and 19.7a, b), 46

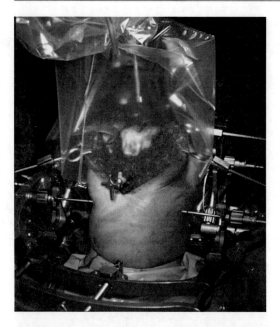

Fig. 19.4 Knee securely fixed with cutting tool and splash guard in place right before femoral milling action commences. The tibial registration cross is still in place at the distal end of the incision (From Konermann W, Haaker R (eds.), Navigation und Robotic in der Gelenkund Wirbelsäulenchirurgie. Berlin, Springer, 2003, with kind permission of Springer Science + Business Media, Inc.)

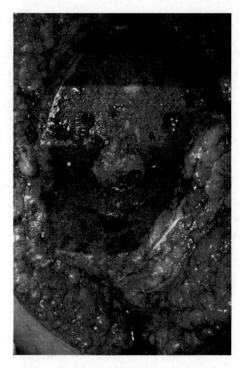

Fig. 19.5 Final tibial and femoral bone surfaces with preserved posterior cruciate ligament (From Konermann W, Haaker R (eds.), Navigation und Robotic in der Gelenkund Wirbelsäulenchirurgie. Berlin, Springer, 2003, with kind permission of Springer Science + Business Media, Inc.)

implants were hybrids (tibia cemented, femur cementless), and seven were completely cementless (Fig. 19.8). The average age of the patients (74 women, 34 men) was 66 years (range, 37–87 years). Patients were clinically evaluated before and after surgery according to the Knee Society Score [10]. All patients were followed up at intervals of 3, 6, 12, 24, and 60 months after surgery. No patients were lost to follow-up.

Before and 2 weeks after surgery, standing long-leg anteroposterior roentgenograms were taken of all patients to control for correct alignment. The mechanical leg axis was measured on these X-ray films and directly compared with the preoperative plan. Data were statistically analyzed by using a two-tailed Student's-test. Statistical significance was assumed at a *p* value smaller than 0.01.

Results

General Observations and Complications

Operating time for the 108 robotic cases averaged 137 min (80–200 min). At discharge, all patients had 90° or greater of flexion. No major adverse events, directly related to the CASPAR system, have been noted. A minor complication occurred in one patient. Due to a defective registration marker, the femoral milling process could not be completed as planned. Full correction was achieved by converting to a manual technique. Three patients had superficial infections at one of the sites where the fiducial marker pins had been fixed to the bone. All infections resolved under conservative management.

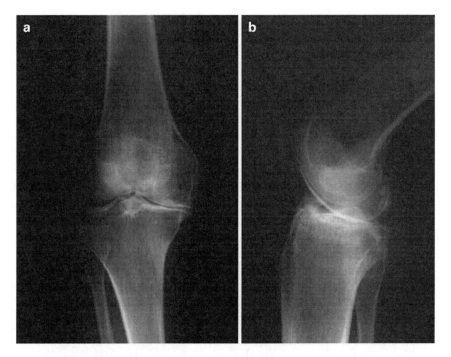

Fig. 19.6 (**a**, **b**) Anteroposterior and lateral X-rays of a patient with medial gonarthrosis before robotic TKA (From Siebert et al., [9] with permission of Elsevier, Inc.)

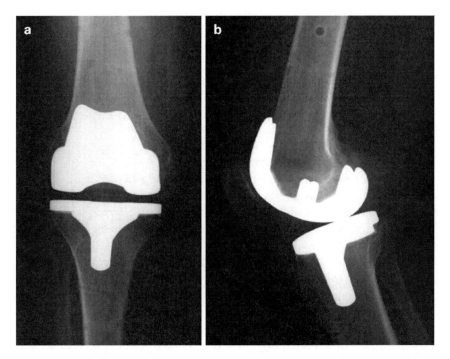

Fig. 19.7 (**a**, **b**) Anteroposterior and lateral X-rays of the same patient after robotic TKA (Search Evolution, Aesculap, Tuttlingen, Germany) (From Siebert et al., [9] with permission of Elsevier, Inc.)

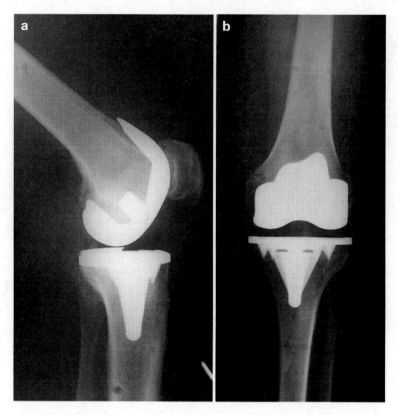

Fig. 19.8 Anteroposterior and lateral X-rays of the same patient after robotic TKA (Genesis, Smith & Nephew, Memphis, TN) (From Siebert et al., [9] with permission of Elsevier, Inc.)

Postoperative Tibiofemoral Alignment

In the computerized preoperative planning procedure, the mechanical axis was routinely corrected to a tibiofemoral angle of 0°. The overall mean difference between the preoperative plan and postoperative result for tibiofemoral alignment was 0.8°, with a standard deviation of 1.0° and a range from 0 to 3°. In addition, the joint line with respect to the position of the femoral and tibial components was in good alignment. In 2004, Decking, with postoperative CT scans, proved the accuracy of this system in all planes, frontal, sagittal, and transverse [11]. The mean tibiofemoral angle in a comparable manual group (NexGen CR Prosthesis, Zimmer, Inc., Warsaw, IN) was 2.6° with a standard deviation of 2.2° and a range from 0 to 7°. Eighteen patients (35%) had a deviation > 3°, with a maximum of 7°.

The exact distribution of varus and valgus deviations of the mechanical axis is shown in Fig. 19.9. The difference in tibiofemoral alignment was highly significant at $p < 0.0001$.

Knee Society Score

The Knee Society Score is divided into the Knee score and the Function score. In each score, the patient can achieve a maximum of 100 points. The difference between the preoperative score and the scores at 12, 24, and 60 months after surgery was significant (Table 19.1). Unfortunately, comorbidity may influence the surgical results, therefore, some patients, especially older patients, rarely achieve the full score and continue loosing functional capabilities as evidenced by slightly lower values at 24 and 60 months postoperatively (Table 19.2).

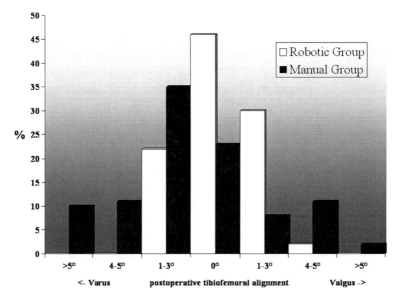

Fig. 19.9 Postoperative tibiofemoral angles of patients after manual and robotic TKA. Measured values show a much broader variation of varus or valgus angles after manual TKA compared with robotic technique ($p < 0.0001$) (From Siebert et al., [9] with permission of Elsevier, Inc.)

Table 19.1 Comparison of knee score preoperative and after 60 months is highly significant in robot-assisted TKA

Knee score	Preoperative	12 months	24 months	60 months
Mean	38.60	87.73	91.59	90.49
Standard deviation	16.36	13.17	11.66	12.09
Number	108	105	96	85

Table 19.2 Comparison of function score preoperatively and after 60 months is highly significant in robot-assisted TKA

Function score	Preoperative	12 months	24 months	60 months
Mean	53.15	81.62	86.72	84.51
Standard deviation	16.04	17.63	17.97	18.39
Number	108	105	96	85

Discussion

Various experimental active and semi-active robotic systems have been developed to improve the accuracy of implant alignment [12]. To our knowledge, this is the only clinical report of robotic TKA in a large series of consecutive patients with a 5-year follow-up.

Our results clearly demonstrate that, after a short learning period, an active robotic system allows the surgeon to execute the preoperative plan with unparalleled accuracy with a mean error below 1° and achieve optimum to very good results regarding tibiofemoral alignment in more than 95% of cases as compared with approximately 65% with manual technique. Aglietti and coworkers reported that the majority of conventionally operated patients end up with a mean valgus angle of 9.6°, ranging from 2 to 16°.[13] Correct tibiofemoral alignment seems to be particularly important because it is generally agreed that axial deviation and imprecise implantation may lead to early loosening of implant components [14–17]. An axial deviation of more than 3° or Maquet's line not passing through the middle third of the implant is considered the most frequent cause of early TKA failure [18–21]. The results of alignment after robotic TKA are not only superior to the results with conventional technique, but also to the results of computer-assisted, navigated TKA. Miehlke and coworkers found that 63% of patients had an acceptable tibiofemoral alignment within the 2° varus/valgus range after navigated TKA. More than 4° of deviation with a maximum error of 7° were observed in almost 7% of the navigated cases [22]. This indicates that although computer-assisted navigation yields superior results to manual technique, it is still inferior to the robotic technique regarding orientation of the prosthetic components. In contrast to the CASPAR system, navigation systems for TKA still depend on intramedullary and extramedullary guides, which might be an important cause for potential errors in axial alignment [23]. Another benefit of the robotic technique might be the accurate planning of the milling track and the type of cutting used. This should result in a reduced risk for injury of ligaments, vessels, and nerves, which are undoubtedly endangered by manually directed oscillating saws. The osseous insertion of the posterior cruciate ligament, for instance, can always be preserved. Implants fit more exactly because the milled surfaces are always precisely flat; a matter of particular importance when cementless systems are used. Finally, the amount of removed bony substance can be minimized, which could facilitate later revision surgery.

There are certain advantages and disadvantages in robot-assisted surgery, as shown in Tables 19.3 and 19.4.

Robotic systems hold great promise in assisting surgeons to perform difficult procedures with a high degree of accuracy and repeatability. Preoperative plans can reliably be translated into clinical reality with the help of a robotic device.

Table 19.3 Advantages of robot-assisted surgery

- Exact preoperative planning and transfer to the robot
- High precision and safety
- Better mechanical axis
- Reduced bone loss
- Exact milling process
- Precision of implantation is less dependent on experience and skill of the surgeon

Table 19.4 Disadvantages of robot-assisted surgery

- Additional cost
- Increased planning time
- Longer operation time
- Soft tissue balancing depending on experience of surgeon
- Additional pins
- Rigid fixation of leg
- Additional CT

The CASPAR system fulfilled these requirements, but had major drawbacks, such as added costs, need for additional surgery, and CT imaging, as well as increased time for preoperative planning and surgery. Being a modified industrial robot that is, e.g., used for computer chip production in clean room environments, the CASPAR system represented quite a cumbersome piece of capital equipment, which, for many hospitals, is difficult to purchase and maintain. Despite excellent clinical results, in particular, in the area of knee arthroplasty, the CASPAR robot did not become a commercial success and the manufacturer stopped production and sales in 2001. Other robotic systems are currently being clinically investigated. Passive robotic systems that leave more control to the surgeon but limit the surgeon's path and range of milling and cutting seem to be ideal candidates for future clinical use, especially when combined with real-time computer navigation [24–26].

References

1. Aglietti P, Buzzi R. Posteriorly stabilised total-condylar knee replacement. J Bone Joint Surg 70B:211, 1988
2. Jeffery RS, Morris RW, Denham RA. Coronal alignment after total knee replacement. J Bone Joint Surg 73B:709, 1991

3. Petersen TL, Engh GA. Radiographic assessment of knee alignment after total knee arthroplasty. J Arthroplasty 3:67, 1988

4. Tew M, Waugh W. Tibiofemoral alignment and the results of knee replacement. J Bone Joint Surg 67B:551, 1985

5. Garg A, Walker PS. Prediction of total knee motion using a three-dimensional computer graphics model. J Biochem 23:45, 1990

6. Kwoh YS, Hou J, Jonckheere EA, Hayati S. A robot with improved absolute positioning accuracy for CT guided stereotactic brain surgery. IEEE Trans Biomed Eng 35(2):153–160, 1998

7. Börner M, Bauer A, Lahmer A. Rechnerunterstützter Robotereinsatz in der Hüftendoprothetik. Orthopäde 26:251–257, 1997

8. Petermann J, Kober R, Heinze, R, Frölich JJ, Heeckt PF, Gotzen L. Computer-assisted planning and robot-assisted surgery in anterior cruciate ligament reconstruction. Oper Tech Orthop 10:50, 2000

9. Siebert W, Mai S, Kober R, Heeckt PF. Technique and first clinical results of robot-assisted total knee replacement. Knee 9:173–180, 2002

10. Insall JN, Dorr LD, Scott R, Scott WN. Rationale of the knee society clinical rating system. Clin Orthop Relat Res 248:13, 1989

11. Decking J, Theis C, Achenbach T, Roth E, Nafe B, Eckhardt A. Robotic total knee arthroplasty: the accuracy of CT-based component placement. Acta Orthop Scand 75:573–579, 2004

12. Howe RD, Matsuoka Y. Robotics for surgery. Annu Rev Biomed Eng 1:211, 1999

13. Aglietti P, Buzzi R, Gaudenzi A. Patellofemoral functional results and complications with the posterior stabilized total condylar knee prosthesis. J Arthroplasty 3:17, 1988

14. Ecker ML, Lotke PA, Sindsor RE, Cella JP. Long-term results after total condylar knee arthroplasty. Significance of radiolucent lines. Clin Orthop Relat Res 216:151, 1987

15. Feng EL, Stuhlberg SD, Wixon RL. Progressive subluxation and polyethylene wear in total knee replacements with flat articular surfaces. Clin Orthop Relat Res 299:60, 1994

16. Laskin RS. Total condylar knee replacement in patients who have rheumatoid arthritis. A ten year follow-up study. J Bone Joint Surg 72A:529, 1990

17. Ritter M, Merbst WA, Keating EM, Faris PM. Radiolucency at the bone-cement interface in total knee replacement. J Bone Joint Surg 76A:60, 1991

18. Goodfellow JW, O'Connor JJ. Clinical results of the Oxford knee. Clin Orthop Relat Res 205:21, 1986

19. Insall JN, Ranawat CS, Aglietti P, Shine J. A comparison of four models of total knee-replacement prosthesis. J Bone Joint Surg 58A:754, 1976

20. Insall JN, Binzzir R, Soudry M, Mestriner LA. Total knee arthroplasty. Clin Orthop Relat Res 192:13, 1985

21. Ranawat CS, Adjei OB. Survivorship analysis and results of total condylar knee arthroplasty. Clin Orthop Relat Res 323:168, 1988

22. Miehlke RK, Clemens U, Kershally S. Computer integrated instrumentation in knee arthroplasty – a comparative study of conventional and computerized technique. Presented at the Fourth Annual North American Program on Computer Assisted Orthopaedic Surgery, Pittsburgh, PA, June 2000

23. Nuño-Siebrecht N, Tanzer M, Bobyn JD. Potential errors in axial alignment using intramedullary instrumentation for total knee arthroplasty. J Arthroplasty 15:228, 2000

24. Shi F, Zhang J, Liu Y, Zhao Z. A hand-eye robotic model for total knee replacement surgery. Med Image Comput Comput Assist Inverv Int Conf Med Image Comput Comput Assist Interv. 8(Pt2):122–30, 2005

25. Adili A. Robot assisted orthopedic surgery. Semin Laparosc Surg 11(2):89, 2004

26. Jakopec M, Harris SJ, Rodriguez y Baena F, Gomes P, Cobb J, Davies BL. The first clinical application of a « hands on » robotic knee surgery system. Comput Aided Surg 6(6):329, 2001

Index